AF572463

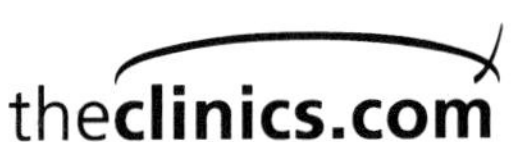

THORACIC SURGERY CLINICS

Management of N2/IIIA Non–Small Cell Lung Cancer

GUEST EDITOR
Mithran S. Sukumar, MD

CONSULTING EDITOR
Mark K. Ferguson, MD

November 2008 • Volume 18 • Number 4

SAUNDERS

An Imprint of Elsevier, Inc.
PHILADELPHIA LONDON TORONTO MONTREAL SYDNEY TOKYO

W.B. SAUNDERS COMPANY
A Division of Elsevier Inc.

1600 John F. Kennedy Boulevard, Suite 1800 • Philadelphia, Pennsylvania 19103-2899

http://www.theclinics.com

THORACIC SURGERY CLINICS
November 2008
Editor: Catherine Bewick

Volume 18, Number 4
ISSN 1547-4127
ISBN-13: 978-1-4160-6362-9
ISBN-10: 1-4160-6362-5

Thoracic Surgery Clinics (ISSN 1547-4127) is published quarterly by Elsevier Inc., 360 Park Avenue South, New York, NY 10010-1710. Months of publication are February, May, August, and November. Business and editorial offices: 1600 John F. Kennedy Boulevard, Suite 1800, Philadelphia, PA 19103-2899. Customer service office: 11830 Westline Industrial Drive, St. Louis, MO 63146. Periodicals postage paid at New York, NY, and additional mailing offices. Subscription prices are $242.00 per year (US individuals), $360.00 per year (US institutions), $121.00 per year (US students), $309.00 per year (Canadian individuals), $455.00 per year (Canadian institutions), $165.00 per year (Canadian and foreign students), $329.00 per year (foreign individuals), and $455.00 per year (foreign institutions). Foreign air speed delivery is included in all *Clinics'* subscription prices. All prices are subject to change without notice. **POSTMASTER:** Send address changes to *Thoracic Surgery Clinics*, Elsevier Journals Customer Service, 11830 Westline Industrial Drive, St. Louis, MO 63146. **Customer Service: 1-800-654-2452 (US and Canada). From outside of the US and Canada, call 1-314-453-7041. Fax: 1-314-453-5170. For print support, e-mail: JournalsCustomerService-usa@elsevier.com. For online support, e-mail: JournalsOnlineSupport-usa@elsevier.com.**

Reprints. For copies of 100 or more, of articles in this publication, please contact Commercial Rights Department, Elsevier Inc., 360 Park Avenue South, New York, NY 10010-1710. Tel: (212) 633-3812; Fax: (212) 462-1935; E-mail: reprints@elsevier.com.

Thoracic Surgery Clinics is covered in *MEDLINE/PubMed (Index Medicus)* and *EMBASE/Excerpta Medica*.

Printed in the United States of America.

CONSULTING EDITOR

MARK K. FERGUSON, MD, Professor of Surgery, Section of Cardiac and Thoracic Surgery, The University of Chicago, Chicago, Illinois

GUEST EDITOR

MITHRAN S. SUKUMAR, MD, Section of General Thoracic Surgery, Oregon Health and Sciences University, Portland Veterans Affairs Medical Center, Portland, Oregon

CONTRIBUTORS

IGOR BRICHKOV, MD, Fellow, Department of Cardiothoracic Surgery, Division of Thoracic Surgery, Albert Einstein College of Medicine, Montefiore Medical Center, Bronx, New York

AYESHA S. BRYANT, MPSH, MD, Assistant Professor, Division of Cardiothoracic Surgery, Department of Surgery; and Department of Epidemiology, University of Alabama at Birmingham School of Public Health, Birmingham, Alabama

ROBERT J. CERFOLIO, MD, FACS, FCCP, Professor of Surgery and Chief, Section of Thoracic Surgery, Division of Cardiothoracic Surgery, Department of Surgery, University of Alabama at Birmingham, Birmingham, Alabama

FRANK DETTERBECK, MD, Department of Surgery, Section of Thoracic Surgery, Yale University, New Haven, Connecticut

LORETTA ERHUNMWUNSEE, MD, Resident, Department of General Surgery, Duke University Medical Center, Durham, North Carolina

THOMAS D'AMICO, MD, Professor, Department of Surgery, Duke University Medical Center, Durham, North Carolina

SHAWN S. GROTH, MD, University of Minnesota, Department of Surgery, Division of General Thoracic and Foregut Surgery, Minneapolis, Minnesota

EDMUND S. KASSIS, MD, Fellow, Department of Thoracic and Cardiovascular Surgery, The University of Texas MD Anderson Cancer Center, Houston, Texas

STEVEN M. KELLER, MD, Professor of Cardiothoracic Surgery and Chief, Department of Cardiothoracic Surgery, Division of Thoracic Surgery, Albert Einstein College of Medicine, Montefiore Medical Center, Bronx, New York

BRIAN E. LALLY, MD, Fox Chase Cancer Center, Department of Radiation Oncology, Philadelphia, Pennsylvania

MICHAEL A. MADDAUS, MD, University of Minnesota, Department of Surgery, Division of General Thoracic and Foregut Surgery, Minneapolis, Minnesota

SHILPEN PATEL, MD, Assistant Professor, Department of Radiation Oncology, Fred Hutchison Cancer Research Center, University of Washington, Seattle, Washington

RACHEL E. SANBORN, MD, Co-Director, Thoracic Oncology Program, Department of Medical Oncology, Providence Portland Medical Center, Portland, Oregon

PAUL SCHIPPER, MD, FACS, FACCP, Assistant Professor, Section of General Thoracic Surgery, Division of Cardiothoracic Surgery, Department of Surgery, Oregon Health and Sciences University, Portland, Oregon

MATT SCHOOLFIELD, MD, Fellow, Section of General Thoracic Surgery, Division of Cardiothoracic Surgery, Department of Surgery, Oregon Health and Sciences University, Portland, Oregon

MITHRAN S. SUKUMAR, MD, Section of General Thoracic Surgery, Oregon Health and Sciences University, Portland Veterans Affairs Medical Center, Portland, Oregon

CHARLES R. THOMAS, Jr., MD, Chair, Department of Radiation Medicine, Oregon Health and Science University, Portland, Oregon

BRANDON H. TIEU, MD, Department of Surgery, Oregon Health and Science University, Portland, Oregon

ARA A. VAPORCIYAN, MD, Associate Professor, Department of Thoracic and Cardiovascular Surgery, The University of Texas MD Anderson Cancer Center, Houston, Texas

BRYAN A. WHITSON, MD, PhD, University of Minnesota, Department of Surgery, Division of General Thoracic and Foregut Surgery, Minneapolis, Minnesota

CONTENTS

FORTHCOMING ISSUES

February 2009

Diseases of the Mediastinum
F. Venuta, *Guest Editor*

May 2009

Surgical and Endoscopic Management of End Stage Emphysema
C. Choong, *Guest Editor*

August 2009

Thoracic Surgery in the Elderly
S. Yang, *Guest Editor*

RECENT ISSUES

August 2008

Frontiers of Minimally Invasive Thoracic Surgery
Gaetano Rocco, MD, FRCS (Ed), FECTS
Guest Editor

May 2008

Hyperhidrosis
Sean C. Grondin, MD, MPH, *Guest Editor*

February 2008

Preoperative Evaluation of Lung Resection Candidates
Alessandro Brunelli, MD, *Guest Editor*

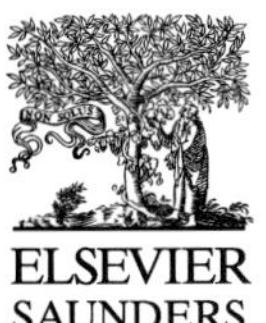
ELSEVIER
SAUNDERS

Thorac Surg Clin 18 (2008) ix

THORACIC
SURGERY
CLINICS

Preface

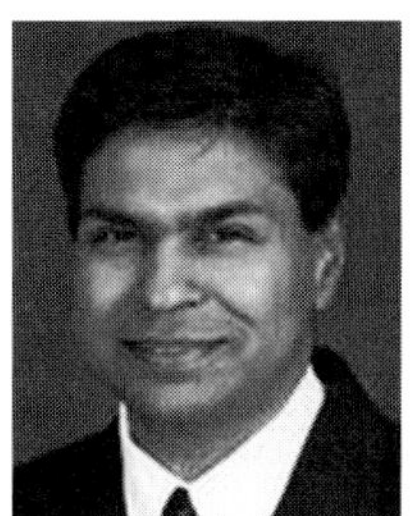

Mithran S. Sukumar, MD
Guest Editor

N2 disease is an interesting and controversial aspect of lung cancer that is evolving as our understanding of the disease progresses. Advances in staging, the use of neoadjuvant therapy, operative planning, and adjuvant therapy require an increasing knowledge of this heterogenous group to provide the appropriate care for these patients.

This issue of *Thoracic Surgery Clinics* is dedicated to fulfilling this requirement.

The articles presented consist of the most up-to-date information on the various aspects of N2 disease, which should allow the practicing thoracic surgeon a better grasp of this aspect of lung cancer.

I wish to thank all the contributing authors for the time taken in presenting their articles in a clear, concise, and meaningful manner. It is my hope that this issue improves our understanding of N2 disease and serves as a practical guide in the care of these patients.

Mithran S. Sukumar, MD
Section of General Thoracic Surgery
Oregon Health and Sciences University
Portland VA Medical Center
3181 SW Sam Jackson Park Road
Portland, OR 97239, USA

E-mail address: sukumarm@ohsu.edu

doi:10.1016/j.thorsurg.2008.08.005

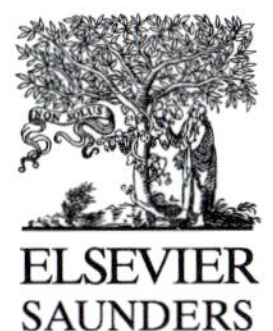

ELSEVIER
SAUNDERS

Thorac Surg Clin 18 (2008) 333–337

THORACIC
SURGERY
CLINICS

Defining N2 Disease in Non–Small Cell Lung Cancer

Edmund S. Kassis, MD, Ara A. Vaporciyan, MD*

Department of Thoracic and Cardiovascular Surgery, The University of Texas MD Anderson Cancer Center, 1515 Holcombe Boulevard, Box 445, Houston, TX 77030, USA

Simply defined, N2 disease in non–small cell lung cancer (NSCLC) is the presence of ipsilateral mediastinal nodal metastases. This definition does little justice to what is in actuality a heterogeneous and challenging patient population. The presence of ipsilateral mediastinal nodal metastases (N2 disease) in NSCLC is a poor prognostic sign. In the series published by Mountain and colleagues [1] from a single institution, 10% of 5319 patients had N2 disease with a 5-year survival of 23%. Recently, the International Association for the Study of Lung Cancer (IASLC) proposed changes to the T, M, and overall stage groupings for patients with NSCLC [2–6]. After analyzing pathologic data from 38,265 patients with NSCLC, Rusch and colleagues identified 11,619 patients with N2 disease and their 5-year survival of 16%. These numbers paint a simplistic view of this prognostic factor. As this article will demonstrate, the definition of N2 disease includes many subgroupings with widely disparate effects on prognosis (Fig. 1).

Many factors contribute to the heterogeneity of this patient population. These include factors related to the involved lymph nodes themselves (location, number, size, and the less clearly defined issue of resectability), the timing of the diagnosis (preresection or clinical versus postresection or pathologic) and the completeness of the mediastinal evaluation (intraoperative sampling versus dissection). Despite extensive studies, no consensus exists regarding these issues. There has been intense interest by numerous investigators to subclassify patients with mediastinal nodal metastases to create more homogeneous populations to improve staging, prognosis, and tailoring of therapy.

In this article we will define and discuss two facets surrounding the definition of N2 disease. The first discussion will center on the issue of clinically staged versus pathologically staged disease (N2 disease identified on final pathologic review of the resected specimen). The second discussion will focus on subsets of N2 disease that have been shown to have a significant impact on prognosis. This discussion will focus primarily on the impact of the number of involved lymph nodes, their location, the number of involved stations, and fixed or unresectable disease.

Clinical versus incidental pathologic N2 disease

The first reports suggesting that patients with clinically detected N2 disease fared worse than patients whose N2 disease was first identified after pulmonary resection were from Pearson and colleagues [7] and Martini and colleagues [8]. In Pearson's study, mediastinoscopy was performed in 76 patients. The 5-year survival for mediastinoscopy-negative but postresection-positive N2 patients was 41% compared with 15% for patients whose N2 disease was identified at mediastinoscopy. Martini and colleagues also demonstrated similar differences with a 5-year survival of 34% versus 9% respectively. These results have been confirmed by recent studies by Andre and colleagues [9] and Vansteenkiste and colleagues [10]. Andre and colleagues reported that the presence of clinical N2 disease and number of involved nodal levels were negative prognostic factors on multivariate analysis. The 5-year survival of patients with clinical (preresection) versus

* Corresponding author.
E-mail address: avaporciyan@mdanderson.org (A.A. Vaporciyan).

1547-4127/08/$ - see front matter. Published by Elsevier Inc.
doi:10.1016/j.thorsurg.2008.07.005

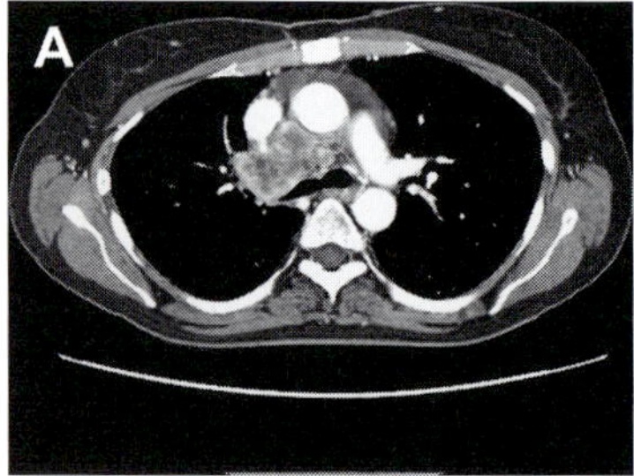

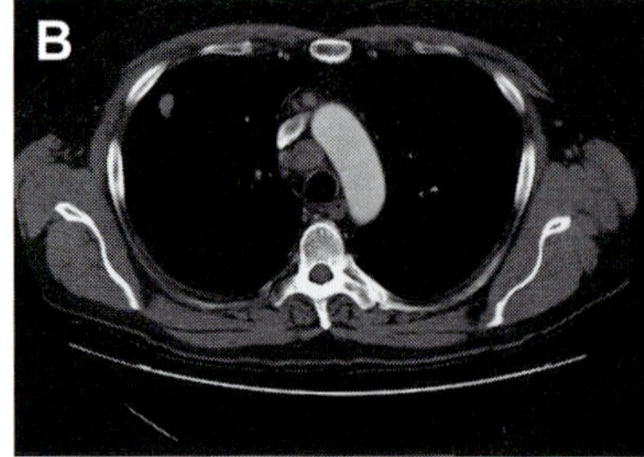

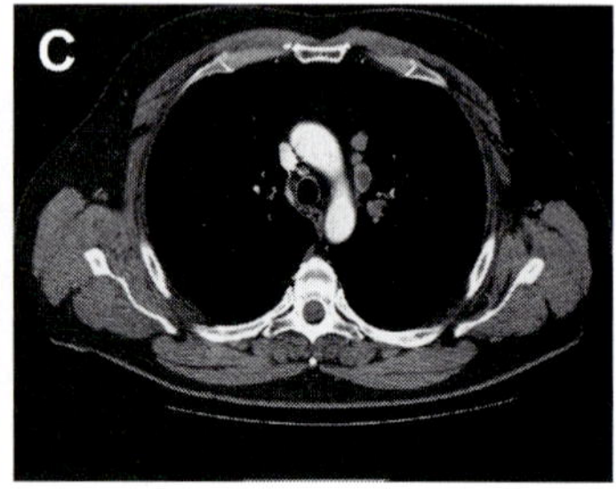

Fig. 1. All three of these patients presented with clinical N2 disease and yet each of them would be approached very differently. Panel A demonstrates a large (>5 cm) "bulky" lesion that clearly compresses the right mainstem bronchus with adherence to the posterior aspect of the superior vena cava. Panel B demonstrated multiple positive stations throughout the ipsilateral mediastinum. Shown here are the enlarged level 4R and level 3A lymph nodes. Panel C depicts a single focus of N2 disease in station 5. Although each of these fits the definition of N2 disease, they each have distinctive effects on prognosis and treatment.

incidental pathologic (postresection) N2 disease was 29% and 7%, respectively. Similarly, Vansteenkiste and colleagues reported that multilevel disease and clinical N2 stage were negative prognostic factors on multivariate analysis. The 5-year survival of their clinically positive N2 versus clinically negative N2 was 32% versus 15%, respectively. These studies suggest that clinical and pathologic N2 disease may be considered distinct entities and may argue for a subclassification of N2 staging. In their discussion, Andre and colleagues argued that since the prognosis of even completely resected clinically identified N2 disease was so poor that this subgroup of patients might be included with stage IIIB patients.

Although intriguing, reclassification is likely not an option since clinical staging is not performed consistently between centers. However, these data do argue for aggressive identification of clinical N2 disease through noninvasive or invasive modalities. These modalities are detailed in this text and elsewhere [11].

While it appears that patients with incidental pathologic N2 disease have a more favorable prognosis then patients with clinically identified N2 disease, the identification of incidental pathologic N2 disease is dependent on careful examination of the mediastinum at the time of resection. Controversy still exists regarding the appropriateness of systematic mediastinal node dissection versus mediastinal node sampling. Although numerous studies have confirmed the improved staging accuracy of node dissection compared with node sampling, very few trials have demonstrated a survival benefit to mediastinal node dissection. Massard and associates [12] studied 208 patients with clinically negative N2 nodes undergoing resection for NSCLC. Patients underwent systematic nodal sampling followed by mediastinal lymph node dissection. Sixty patients had pathologic N2 disease with 25 patients having multilevel disease and 24 patients with skip metastases. Of the 60 patients with N2 disease, lymph node sampling identified only 31 (52%). Additionally, sampling identified multilevel disease in only 10 (40%) of 25 of patients. The overall sensitivity, specificity, positive predictive value, and negative predictive value for sampling was 51.6%, 100.0%, 100.0%, and 83.6%, respectively. No comment was made on rate of complication or overall survival. Similar findings have been reported by Wu and colleagues [13] and Keller and colleagues [14]. Wu and colleagues [13] randomized 532 patients to mediastinal sampling or dissection. Mediastinal dissection identified more patients with N2 disease than did nodal sampling. Keller and colleagues [14] studied 373 patients with either N1 or N2 disease. A total of 187 patients underwent mediastinal sampling and 186 underwent complete mediastinal nodal dissection. When N2 disease was present, multilevel disease was found in 30% of patients undergoing nodal dissection compared with only 12% of patients undergoing sampling. These studies suggest that a complete dissection will allow more accurate staging of patients with N2 disease. The randomized study by Wu and colleagues even demonstrated improved survival with dissection. Certainly the identification of N2 disease would justify the delivery of adjuvant chemotherapy, which may have been withheld if sampling had been employed. The subsequent benefit of adjuvant chemotherapy [15] would be potentially lost without a complete dissection.

Further data regarding dissection versus sampling will be derived from the recent completion of a multi-institutional trial sponsored by the American College of Surgeons Oncology Group. This trial (ACOSOG Z0030) randomized patients intraoperatively to dissection versus sampling and is adequately powered to address the issue of a survival advantage. Allen and colleagues [16] have already presented the initial results regarding the morbidity and mortality associated with the separate techniques. While node dissection resulted in greater intraoperative blood loss, operative time, and chest tube drainage, it was not associated with an increased length of stay or rate of postoperative complications. The survival data are still maturing.

Subsets of N2 disease

Although the presence of N2 disease is clearly a negative prognostic sign, there are subsets of patients that deserve special attention. Both favorable and unfavorable subsets have been suggested and many are summarized in Table 1. Those factors with supporting data, such as the impact of single-level versus multilevel N2 disease, the patterns of nodal spread, and the importance of fixed or unresectable nodal metastases will be discussed here.

Single versus multistation disease

Riquet and associates [17] recently published data on 586 patients with N2 disease who underwent curative resection. In this study, patients with single-level N2 disease had a superior 5-year survival compared with patients with multilevel N2 disease, 28.5% versus 17.2% respectively.

Table 1
Commonly cited factors that influence the impact of N2 disease

Favorable	Unfavorable
Single-station involvement	Multistation involvement
Single node	Multiple nodes
Microscopic disease	Extracapsular extension
Station 5 or 6	Station 4L or 9
Small-volume disease	Bulky disease
	Fixed (invasion of mediastinal structures)
	Skip metastasis

In contrast to other studies, the histology of the primary tumor, the location of the primary tumor, the location of involved lymph nodes [18,19], the presence of capsular rupture [20,21], or the number of metastatic lymph nodes [22,23] were not found to influence survival. Interestingly, the 5-year survival in patients with skip metastases was better than those without skip metastases, 38% versus 23.3% respectively. Surprisingly, the presence of micrometastases in N2 nodes was an indicator of a worse prognosis. This is in contrast to other studies demonstrating an improved prognosis in patients with micrometastatic disease [9].

Casali and colleagues [24] analyzed data from 183 patients with pathologically proven N2 NSCLC. Multilevel N2 disease was associated with a 5-year survival of 14.7% compared with 23.8% in patients with single-level disease. Andre and colleagues [9] studied 686 patients with histologically proven N2 disease who underwent surgical resection. In this study, 38% of patients had involvement of multiple nodal levels. In patients with pathologic N2 disease, multiple-level involvement was found on multivariate analysis to be a negative prognostic factor with a 5-year survival of 11% compared with 34% for single-level disease. The survival of patients with clinical N2 disease and multiple-level involvement had a 5-year survival of 3%. Similarly, Ichinose and colleagues [25] reported a 5-year survival of 43% in 209 patients with single-level N2 disease compared with 17% in patients with multilevel disease. These investigators probed further and examined the impact of single- versus multiple-station disease relative to the site of the primary tumor. The benefit of a single-station involvement was seen in every lobe except left lower lobe tumors. For this site there was no advantage to single-station N2 disease.

Patterns of nodal involvement

Several articles in the past decade have demonstrated that not only are the number of lymph nodes and nodal levels important prognostically but that the pattern of nodal spread with relation to the primary tumor also impacts survival [18,19]. In the manuscript by Keller and associates [26], 373 patients received surgery for NSCLC with complete intraoperative lymph node assessment. Of these, 223 had pathologic N2 disease. The median survival of patients with N1 disease was significantly better than the patients with either multilevel or single-level N2 disease. Unlike other investigators, they found no significant difference between single- and multilevel N2 disease. Interestingly, there was no difference in survival for patients with left upper lobe tumors and either N1 or single-level N2 disease. Of the 49 patients with left upper lobe tumors and single-level N2 disease 43 had metastases in stations 5 or 6. This suggests that isolated metastases in these stations for upper lobe tumor may behave similarly to N1 metastases. Skip metastases to N2 nodes in absence of N1 nodes also fared better than those patients without skip metastases. This benefit was isolated only to those patients with left upper lobe tumors.

Nakanishi and colleagues presented similar findings with a survival benefit seen in patients with a station 5 or 6 node versus nodal involvement anywhere else. However, this survival advantage was lost when multiple stations were involved.

Bulky or unresectable N2 disease

This group of patients is the least defined but most commonly cited prognostic factor in assessing N2 disease. For many clinical trials involving surgery in patients with N2 disease, this factor defined the subgroup that would be eligible. However, the definition was not always clearly stated being primarily determined by the evaluating surgeon. The true definition of this subset is likely an amalgam of all the factors that have already been presented. "Bulky" disease may refer to a single giant node (>5 cm) or multistation involvement. As previously discussed, clinically evident multistation disease is a very poor prognostic sign and avoidance of surgery for this subset is very appropriate. The term "unresectable" may also have numerous interpretations. One interpretation, that of fixed disease, most likely refers to nodal disease that has invaded mediastinal structures. However, other interpretations of this term may include multistation disease or large, greater than 5 cm, disease. Considering the heterogeneity of N2 disease, every effort should be made to avoid these sorts of ambiguous terms. It is hoped that in the future, clinical trails will define their eligibility criteria to carefully identify the subgroups of N2 disease that will be enrolled.

Miscellaneous

Other subgroups of N2 disease have been suggested, both favorable and unfavorable (see Table 1). The presence of capsular rupture [20,21], the number of metastatic lymph nodes [22,23], N2 disease presenting as a skip metastases, and N2 disease presenting as micrometastatic disease [9] have all been suggested in various reports to influence the survival of N2-positive patients. It is likely that additional subgroups have and will be suggested as improvements in imaging and evaluation continue.

Summary

In summary, patients with N2 disease constitute a heterogeneous population with differing treatments and prognoses. Subtleties in the presentation, method of diagnosis, extent of nodal involvement, and patterns of nodal involvement must be taken into consideration to determine prognosis and optimal therapy. Is the patient with an incidental, pathologically identified, single focus of mediastinal disease the same as the patient with clinically identified multilevel bulky unresectable disease? Clearly not, although both patients share a similar stage, grouping the data presented here clearly demonstrate that these patients differ considerable in their prognosis and in their treatment. The current staging system attempts at assigning a single unifying definition of N2 fails to take into account the numerous subtleties inherent in this patient population. Although it is unlikely that N2 disease will be subclassified to any significant extent, some of these factors may eventually find themselves into a modern revision of our current staging system. For now, the upcoming IASLC revisions to the Union Internationale Contre le Cancer (UICC) staging system will not alter the definitions of nodal disease or add distinct subsets. Therefore, it is imperative that physicians evaluating and treating patients with N2 disease recognize and appreciate the influence of these subtle differences in presentation. Decision making surrounding the treatment of N2-positive patients will continue to remain complex as long as the definition of the disease remains heterogeneous.

References

[1] Mountain CF. Revisions in the international system for staging lung cancer. Chest 1997;111:1710–7.

[2] Tomlins SA, Laxman B, Dhanasekaran SM, et al. Distinct classes of chromosomal rearrangements create oncogenic ETS gene fusions in prostate cancer. Nature 2007;448:595–9.

[3] Wrana JL, Attisano L. The Smad pathway. Cytokine Growth Factor Rev 2000;11:5–13.

[4] Miyazawa K, Shinozaki M, Hara T, et al. Two major Smad pathways in TGF-beta superfamily signalling. Genes Cells 2002;7:1191–204.

[5] Han HJ, Russo J, Kohwi Y, et al. SATB1 reprogrammes gene expression to promote breast tumour growth and metastasis. Nature 2008;452:187–93.

[6] Meyerson M. Cancer: broken genes in solid tumours. Nature 2007;448:545–6.

[7] Pearson FG, Delarue NC, Ilves R, et al. Significance of positive superior mediastinal nodes identified at mediastinoscopy in patients with resectable cancer of the lung. J Thorac Cardiovasc Surg 1982;83(1): 1–11.

[8] Martini N, Flehinger BJ, Zaman MB, et al. Results of resection in non-oat cell carcinoma of the lung with mediastinal lymph node metastases. Ann Surg 1983;198(3):386–97.

[9] Andre F, Grunenwald D, Pignon JP, et al. Survival of patients with resected N2 non-small-cell lung cancer: Evidence for a subclassification and implications. J Clin Oncol 2000;18:2981–9.

[10] Vansteenkiste JF, Deleyn PR, Deneffe GJ, et al. Survival and prognostic factors in resected N2 non-small cell lung cancer: a study of 140 cases. Ann Thorac Surg 1997;63:1441–50.

[11] Kim ES, Bosquee L. The importance of accurate lymph node staging in early and locally advanced non-small cell lung cancer: an update on available techniques. J Thorac Oncol 2007;2:S59–67.

[12] Massard G, Ducrocq X, Kochetkova EA, et al. Sampling or node dissection for intraoperative staging of lung cancer: a multicentric cross-sectional study. Eur J Cardiothorac Surg 2006;30:164–7.

[13] Wu Y, Huang Z, Wand S. A randomized trial of systematic nodal dissecton in resectable non-small cell lung cancer. Lung Cancer 2003;36:1–6.

[14] Keller SM, Adak S, Wagner H, et al. Mediastinal lymph node dissection improves survival in patients with stages II and IIIa non-small cell lung cancer. Eastern Cooperative Oncology Group. Ann Thorac Surg 2000;70:358–65.

[15] Pignon JP, Tribodet H, Scagliotti GV, et al. Lung Adjuvant Cisplatin Evaluation (LACE): a pooled analysis of five randomized clinical trials including 4,584 patients. J Clin Oncol 2006;24:366S.

[16] Allen MS, Darling GE, Pechet TT, et al. Morbidity and mortality of major pulmonary resections in patients with early-stage lung cancer: Initial results of the randomized, prospective ACOSOG Z0030 trial. Ann Thorac Surg 2006;81:1013–9.

[17] Riquet M, Bagan P, Le Pimpec Barthes F, et al. Completely resected non-small cell lung cancer: reconsidering prognostic value and significance of N2 metastases. Ann Thorac Surg 2007;84:1818–24.

[18] Maggi G, Casadio C, Cianci R, et al. Results of surgical resection of stage-IIIA (N2) non-small-cell lung-cancer, according to the site of the mediastinal metastases. Int Surg 1993;78:213–7.

[19] Nakanishi R, Osaki T, Nakanishi K, et al. Treatment strategy for patients with surgically discovered N2 stage IIIA non-small cell lung cancer. Ann Thorac Surg 1997;64:342–8.

[20] Cybulsky I, Lanza L, Ryan M, et al. Prognostic significance of computed tomography in resection N2 lung cancer. Ann Thorac Surg 1992;54:533–7.

[21] Suemasu K, Naruke T. Prognostic significance of extranodal cancer invasion of mediastinal lymph nodes in lung cancer. Jpn J Cancer Res 1982;12(2): 207–12.

[22] Hata E, Hayakawa K, Miyamoto H, et al. Rationale for extended lymphadenectomy for lung-cancer. Theor Surg 1990;5:19–25.

[23] Miller DL, McManus KG, Allen MS, et al. Results of surgical resection in patients with N2 non-small cell lung cancer. Ann Thorac Surg 1994;57:1095–100.

[24] Casali C, Stefania A, Natalia P, et al. Prognostic factors in surgically resected N2 non-small cell lung cancer: the importance of patterns of mediastinal lymph nodes metastases. European Journal of Cardiothoracic Surgery 2005;28:33–8.

[25] Ichinose Y, Kato H, Koike T, et al. Completely resected stage IIIA non-small cell lung cancer: the significance of primary tumor location and N2 station. J Thorac Cardiovasc Surg 2001;122:803–8.

[26] Keller SM, Vangel MG, Wagner H, et al. Prolonged survival in patients with resected non-small cell lung cancer and single-level N2 disease. J Thorac Cardiovasc Surg 2004;128:130–7.

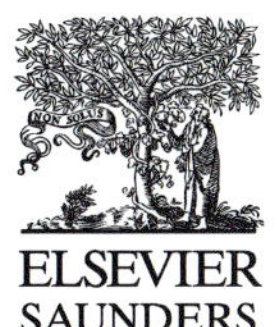
ELSEVIER
SAUNDERS

Thorac Surg Clin 18 (2008) 339–347

THORACIC
SURGERY
CLINICS

Detection of Occult N2 Disease with Molecular Techniques

Loretta Erhunmwunsee, MD[a], Thomas A. D'Amico, MD[b,*]

[a]*Department of General Surgery, Duke University Medical Center, Box 3443, Durham, NC 27710, USA*
[b]*Department of Surgery, Duke University Medical Center, Box 3496, Duke South, White Zone, Room 3589, Durham, NC 27710, USA*

Lung cancer is the number one cancer killer in the United States, responsible for more deaths than breast cancer, colon cancer, pancreatic cancer, and prostate cancer combined [1]. Accurate determination of nodal status is critical to the staging of patients with non–small cell lung cancer (NSCLC), both in terms of assessment of prognosis [2–4] and assignment of therapy [5]. For patients with resectable lung cancer, the finding of N1 or N2 involvement after surgery is an indication for adjuvant therapy; for those with N2 disease found preoperatively, induction therapy followed by surgery or definitive chemotherapy and radiation therapy is favored [5]. Thus, the ability to accurately assess nodal disease is one of the cornerstones of staging for patients with NSCLC.

Staging by radiologic imaging, such as computed tomography (CT) and positron emission tomography (PET), is routinely performed to determine nodal metastasis. For patients with potentially resectable NSCLC, confirmation through tissue diagnosis is imperative in patients with suspicious nodes, however, because radiologic examination of nodes is not 100% accurate. CT scans are known to have both a low specificity and sensitivity in the detection of mediastinal metastases. Wallace and colleagues [6] found that in the detection of mediastinal nodes, CT had a sensitivity of 87% and a specificity of 32%. PET scans have been reported to have a diagnostic accuracy of 81.6% and a positive predictive value of only 49.3% when detecting metastatic nodes in lung cancer [7–9]. Thus, mediastinoscopy with biopsy and histologic assessment is the standard for staging mediastinal lymph nodes [5,10]. However, microscopic involvement (occult N2 disease) may be missed by routine pathologic techniques. In this review, the methods of assessment of microscopic (occult) N2 disease are discussed, including standard pathologic techniques and emerging molecular strategies.

* Corresponding author.
E-mail address: damic001@mc.duke.edu (T.A. D'Amico).

Hematoxylin and eosin staining

Because nodal status is such a strong prognostic factor, it is imperative that accurate nodal staging is performed. Currently, the standard for detecting nodal involvement is via histologic techniques. Hematoxylin and eosin (H&E) staining is a histologic technique performed on sections of paraffin-embedded or frozen nodes retrieved from mediastinoscopy or from the lung cancer resection specimen. Hematoxylin is a basic dye that colors basophilic structures (such as nucleic acids) blue or purple, whereas eosin is acidic and colors eosinophilic structures (such as proteins) pink. The H&E technique allows visualization of abnormal cells and nuclei [11]. Metaplastic and dysplastic features are readily observed and diagnosis of nodal metastasis is made. The technique includes rehydration of the slides by serial dips in xylene and graded ethanols into distilled water. The slides are then dipped in hematoxylin, rinsed in water and again dipped in eosin. They are lastly dehydrated and mounted. Once stained, the slides are viewed with a microscope. H&E staining is

1547-4127/08/$ - see front matter
doi:10.1016/j.thorsurg.2008.07.001

standard for nodal metastatic diagnosis and has a sensitivity of 92% to 99% [11].

H&E is most accurate when multiple serial sections—typically 1 to 30 μm thick—are stained. Serial sectioning enhances the evaluation of the tissue, while increasing the time to complete it. Although H&E is the current standard for mediastinal nodal metastasis evaluation, other methods are currently studied [5].

Cytology

Cytologic assessment of cancer cells is frequently performed for many tumor types; however, in the evaluation of lung tumors, cytologic evaluation of lymph nodes is not routine. Okubo and colleagues [12] studied the use of cytology in the examination of nodal metastasis in lung cancer, assessing regional nodes excised from 151 patients via standard mediastinoscopy or thoracoscopy. The nodes were then bisected, imprinted on a glass slide, fixed, and Papanicolaou stain used. The remainder of the node was used for H&E assessment. The sensitivity, specificity, accuracy, positive predictive value, and negative predictive value of the cytologic technique (95.7%, 100.0%, 99.4%, 100.0% and 99.3%, respectively) compared favorable with the evaluation by H&E (87.1%, 100.0%, 98.1%, 100.0%, and 97.7%, respectively). The authors suggest that cytologic examination is no less helpful than histologic examination for the detection of nodal metastasis but provides the benefit of speed and reduced cost. Clarke and colleagues [13] favor cytology examination to frozen section analysis as well. Their study also revealed high sensitivity and specificity (96.6% and 100,0% respectively) and faster times (2 minutes for cytologic evaluation versus 11 minutes with frozen section). Cytologic detection may have a place in lung cancer staging, especially in centers where frozen section techniques are not readily available or if even faster detection or lower costs are important to the team.

Immunohistochemistry

Immunohistochemistry (IHC) is routinely used in laboratory research and is becoming increasingly more popular in tumor detection. This technique is based on antigen-antibody relationships: a primary antibody detects the antigen (tumor marker) of choice and a secondary antibody that is conjugated to a color-producing enzyme or tagged with a fluorescent molecule detects the primary antibody [14,15]. The emitted color or fluorescence signifies the presence of the specific antigen.

When metastatic nodal disease is being evaluated, the antigen targeted must be one that is present in cancer cells but absent in the normal, noncancerous lymph node. Cytokeratin antigens are intermediate filaments present in the cytoplasm of epithelial tissue and epithelial cancers. They are typically absent in normal lymph nodes and thus are routinely targeted in the detection of epithelial cancers. There are a number of cytokeratin proteins and different combinations of them are present in various epithelial organs. This technique has been used in the staging of other malignancies, such as breast cancer and colorectal cancer. Cote and colleagues [16] studied lymph nodes from 736 patients with breast cancer in Trial V of the International Ludwig Breast Cancer Study. In this study, 7% of the lymph nodes were positive for metastases using the H&E method of detection, whereas IHC, using antibodies to cytokeratin targets (AE-1 and CAM 5.2), found that 20% of the lymph nodes had occult metastases. The authors concluded that single-section immunohistochemistry was more sensitive than the serial-section H&E method in detecting occult lymph node metastases in tumors of all histologic subtypes.

Passlick and colleagues [17] compared IHC and H&E techniques by obtaining lymph nodes from 72 patients with completely resected NSCLC. All of the patients were assessed by H&E and found to be free of nodal metastasis. They then performed IHC on the nodes using BerEP4, a monoclonal antibody against two glycoproteins that are present on the surface and cytoplasm of epithelial cells. The antibody found 15% of the nodes to harbor occult metastases.

Vollmer and colleagues [18] retrieved 825 lymph nodes from 193 patients with NSCLC in the Cancer and Leukemia Group B (CALGB) Trial 9761. Eligible patients had mediastinal nodes that were less than 1 cm by CT scan and nodes sampled by mediastinoscopy that were histologically negative. H&E discovered 18 positive lymph nodes, whereas IHC using the AE1/3 anticytokeratin antibodies detected 45 positive lymph nodes, of which 28 of the lymph nodes had occult metastases only. Nine of these 28 positive nodes were in N1 stations and 18 were in N2 stations. This study concluded that IHC with AE1/3 anticytokeratin antibodies detects greater than twice as many positive regional lymph nodes as does H&E staining and found that the foci of tumor that IHC detects are significantly smaller than those detected by H&E staining.

The above studies suggest that IHC is more sensitive than H&E in detecting metastatic involvement in regional nodes. Thus occult metastases hidden from H&E can be detected via IHC using antibodies to epithelial antigens. There is considerable evidence that IHC is more sensitive than H&E but is immunohistochemical detection of occult cancer cells significant? Is there evidence that occult metastases are responsible for lower survival or increased recurrence?

Clinical significance of micrometastatic disease

Although IHC and other techniques may improve the ability to detect occult N2 disease, which may increase the accuracy of prognostic stratification, there is not a consensus as to whether this leads to better treatment strategies and outcomes. Kubuschok and associates [19] prospectively studied 117 NSCLC patients with T1-4 N0-2 M0 after complete resection. In this study, 565 of these patients' nodes were histologically negative for disease. Using IHC with the BerEP4 antibody, they found 21.6% of the nodes to have occult metastases. These patients were followed for 5 years and results showed that patients with occult metastases had reduced disease-free and overall survival. The report also revealed that occult metastasis corresponded to 2.7 times increased risk for tumor relapse and 2.5 times increased risk for shorter survival compared with patients without such cells. Patients without any evidence of nodal involvement had an overall survival rate of 78% [19]. Coello and colleagues [20] recently published a review of the literature and found that occult metastases in stage I NSCLC were associated with increased recurrence and death and suggested that the survival of stage I patients who suffered from occult metastases detected by IHC was similar to those with overt disease. Subsequently, Riquet and colleagues [21] retrospectively evaluated the survival of patients with N2 disease and found that patients with micrometastatic disease had worse outcomes than those with overt disease. Over the course of 9 years, they performed mediastinoscopy on 586 patients found to have N2 disease (25% of all of their patients). These patients were classified into three groups: those with micrometastatic disease (53 patients), those with nonbulky nodal disease (207 patients), and those with bulky nodal disease (126 patients). When only one mediastinal nodal basin was involved, patients with nonbulky disease had a 5-year survival of 32.5% and a median survival of 30 months. Those with bulky disease had a 5-year survival of 27.6% and a median survival of 23 months, whereas those with micrometastatic disease had a 5-year survival of only 16.6% and median survival of 23 months. They explain their results by suggesting that micrometastases may be associated with higher tumor aggressiveness, leading to worse outcomes.

Although many studies suggest that occult disease negatively affects outcome, Marchevsky and colleagues [22] report that patients with micrometastatic disease have the same survival as those without nodal involvement. They performed H&E and IHC on the lymph nodes of 60 patients with NSCLC and followed them for a minimum of 5 years. They classified metastases as isolated tumor cells if the metastases were less than 0.2 mm and classified them as micrometastatic if the metastases were between 0.2 mm and 2.0 mm. They found no significant survival differences between patients with pN0, isolated tumor cells, and pN1 with micrometastatic disease. They also found no instances of micrometastatic disease in their 16 pN2 patients and none of their 11 pN1 patients were upstaged. They conclude that IHC can detect isolated tumor cells in histologically negative nodes. But they suggest that many of these tumor-harboring nodes are seen in patients with other positive pN1 and pN2 lymph nodes and thus the presence of the occult metastases does not lead to a stage change [22].

Improved detection of occult disease in mediastinal nodes continues to be studied. IHC augments histologic techniques but is not ideal. The targeted antigen may not be present in very poorly differentiated tumors and thus not detected by IHC. Also, nonepithelial cells can potentially express cytokeratin proteins, which could increase the false-positive rate of detection. Efforts are now under way to find more accurate means of nodal metastases detection using molecular techniques.

Reverse transcriptase polymerase chain reaction

Reverse transcriptase polymerase chain reaction (RT-PCR) is a technique used to determine the presence of specific gene expression by amplifying the expression of RNA. A reverse transcriptase enzyme (an RNA-dependent DNA polymerase) works on an mRNA template, using primers and deoxynucleotides to create a complementary DNA (cDNA). A DNA polymerase enzyme is then used to amplify the cDNA during the polymerase chain reaction phase. Nested RT-PCR is another method used to further increase the sensitivity of RT-PCR. During this technique, a small amount of the product from the primary RT-PCR is used as a template for a secondary round of PCR amplification. New primers are used to avoid amplification of artifacts that have been created during the primary amplification [23]. Real-time or quantitative PCR is another type of reaction that amplifies the cDNA using a fluoropore or dye that binds to the double-stranded product. The color emitted is read at the end of each PCR cycle, giving the relative amount of product (DNA) produced. With this method, a real time determination of the quantity of genetic product can be ascertained.

Both quantitative and nonquantitative RT-PCR techniques are being explored in cancer detection, as there is evidence that RT-PCR is a more sensitive and specific detector of gene-specific cancer cells than are H&E or IHC. RT-PCR can detect mRNA in poorly differentiated tumors when tissue-specific proteins are not expressed. Also RT-PCR can detect one cancer cell among 10^{6-7} normal cells, versus IHC, which can detect one cancer cell in 10^{4-5} normal cells [24]. And with RT-PCR there is the ability to analyze the entire specimen, decreasing sampling errors.

Assessment of carcinoembryonic antigen with reverse transcriptase polymerase chain reaction

In IHC, targeting the correct antigen with a specific antibody is paramount to precise detection. In RT-PCR, starting with the correct mRNA is crucial to successful analysis. Many investigators are working to determine which gene transcript best finds occult nodal metastases and thus should be targeted in RT-PCR. One such potential marker is the carcinoembryonic antigen (CEA), a glycoprotein that is involved with cell adhesion. It is most known for serving as a serum marker of colorectal cancer recurrence, as elevation of its levels after resection of the tumor corresponds to recurrence. Elevated serum CEA levels are also associated with benign disease like pancreatitis, ulcerative colitis, and cirrhosis. CEA is routinely measured in the serum of patients with cancer but it is also present in the tumor site as well. Its presence in cancer tissue makes it a natural presumptive marker for detection of nodal metastases.

Mori and colleagues [25] used RT-PCR of CEA mRNA to detect micrometastatic disease in 117 nodes from breast, esophageal, gastric, and colon cancer patients. They found that CEA mRNA was expressed in normal mucosal tissue but not in the lymph nodes of normal controls. They detected occult metastases by histology in 26% of the nodes, whereas RT-PCR found amplification of CEA in 66% of the nodes. D'Cunha and colleagues [26] were the first to use quantitative RT-PCR to detect CEA mRNA in the regional nodes of NSCLC patients. They studied 232 lymph nodes from 53 stage I (clinically node negative) patients who were completely resected and found that 25.4% of the nodes were positive for CEA mRNA. These results corresponded to a 56.6% upstaging rate in their 53 patients.

Nosotti and colleagues [24] used quantitative RT-PCR of CEA mRNA to detect micrometastatic disease in 261 lymph nodes from 44 surgically resected clinically stage I NSCLC patients. They followed these patients for a mean of 22.5 months. Of the 261 nodes, 35 (13.4%) had CEA mRNA levels that were higher than those detected in control lymph nodes and were considered positive for micrometastatic disease. They also found that there was less cancer recurrence in patients with lymph nodes negative for CEA mRNA.

The above reports provide evidence that RT-PCR of CEA mRNA detects metastatic nodal disease and can provide prognostic information in NSCLC patients. Bostick and coworkers [27], however, evaluated the potential of specific mRNA markers to detect micrometastatic disease by RT-PCR. They found that CEA mRNA was expressed in the blood of 46% of their 16 patients without cancer. They also sampled three nodes from noncancerous patients and CEA was expressed in three of three of the nodes by RT-PCR. They conclude that the low specificity of CEA prevents it from having diagnostic value as a detector of micrometastatic disease. Wallace and colleagues [28] also found high levels of CEA in their negative controls' lymph nodes. The detection of CEA mRNA more sensitively discovers occult metastases to regional nodes but its low specificity detected by some studies may prevent it from having strong clinical utility. Larger analyses are necessary to further evaluate this marker.

MUC1

The MUC1 gene encodes a mucin cell surface glycoprotein that is expressed in most epithelial tissues, including lung, and is overexpressed in many epithelial cancers. MUC1 was the first marker to be used in the detection of metastatic NSCLC [28]. Salerno and colleagues [29] recently used nested RT-PCR to detect MUC1 mRNA in 28 patients with NSCLC. They found 34% of the nodes retrieved from histologically negative stage I patients demonstrated MUC1 mRNA positivity. In this study, 33% of stage II histologically cancer-negative nodes were positive for MUC1 mRNA and 44% of their IIIa nodes were positive. None of the lymph nodes from patients with benign disease expressed MUC1 mRNA. They then performed IHC with antibodies against MUC1 on 20 nodes that were found to be MUC1 mRNA positive by RT-PCR. Only 9 of the 20 nodes were IHC positive, suggesting that RT-PCR is more sensitive. According to these results, 10 of 23 patients would have a change in stage with a subsequent lowering of the expected survival rate.

Some have criticized MUC1 for being too ubiquitous in expression to be useful in micrometastatic disease detection [27,28,30]. Bostick and colleagues [27] discovered MUC1 expression in 46% of the blood of their noncancerous patients and in 100% of their normal lymph nodes, whereas Saintigny and colleagues [30] found MUC1 expression in three of four noncancerous patients' peripheral blood mononuclear cells. They hypothesized that the cross-reactivity may have occurred by contamination during venipuncture of the sample by skin sebaceous, sweat glands, or monocytes, which all express MUC1 mRNA. This study concluded that MUC1 mRNA detection should not be considered a reliable marker for the detection of micrometastatic cells. In light of the variability of these results from the above noted studies, MUC1 too will need further, more powerful studies to determine its effectiveness as a marker of NSCLC nodal metastasis.

KS1/4

Another potential marker for RT-PCR detection of nodal metastasis is KS1/4, also called TACSTD1, EPCAM, EGP-2, GA-733-2, and MIC-18. Wallace and colleagues [28] performed RT-PCR on the mediastinal nodes from 87 NSCLC patients without radiological evidence of metastases. They found that KS1/4 was overexpressed in 25 of 27 (93%) cytology-positive mediastinal lymph nodes but had very little expression in their 17 healthy control patients. Xi and coworkers [31] also found that KS1/4 (called TACSTD1 in this study) was a useful marker for NSCLC metastasis. They screened numerous potential markers via analysis of expression in 6 primary NSCLC and 10 benign lymph nodes. Those that had high expression in the primary tumors and low expression in the benign lymph nodes went through a secondary screen, which was performed on 21 primary tumors, 21 histologically positive lymph nodes, and 21 benign lymph nodes. Eight markers stood out and were then validated and used to identify occult metastases in 462 nodes from 68 patients with NSCLC. These values were compared with their respective expression in 30 benign nodes analyzed in the previous screening and validation phases. They report a 7.9-fold difference between the positive and benign nodal expression of TACSTD1 and found that it had a sensitivity of 100% in detecting tumor in the 21 histologically positive NSCLC nodes.

Using RT-PCR detection of KS1/4, Mitas and colleagues [32] also found overexpression of KS1/4 in mediastinal nodes. They performed the RT-PCR on nine cancer-containing mediastinal lymph nodes retrieved by endoscopic ultrasound with fine-needle aspiration and on negative control lymph nodes. KS1/4 was overexpressed in nine of nine positive lymph nodes, giving it a sensitivity of 100%. It also was not expressed in any of the negative control lymph nodes and thus KS1/4 exhibited 100% specificity as well.

CK-19

Analysis of cytokeratin expression, discussed above using IHC, may be improved by more advanced techniques. CK-19 is found in many epithelial tissues of visceral organs, such as the bladder, gallbladder, and colon and in many adenocarcinomas and squamous cell carcinomas, but it is not detected in the epidermis or found in normal lymph nodes [33]. Saintigny and coworkers [30] evaluated CK19 expression by quantitative RT-PCR in 43 NSCLC samples, in 94 mediastinal lymph nodes (84 of which were histologically negative), in blood mononuclear cells from 29 healthy volunteers and in 17 benign lymph nodes (nonmediastinal). CK-19 mRNA was not detected in the 17 benign lymph nodes and blood cells from the 29 healthy donors. In the 10 histologically positive mediastinal lymph nodes, CK19 mRNA was detected seven times and was detected in 2 of the 84 histologically negative nodes. They concluded that CK19 mRNA detection is a reliable marker for carcinomatous cells with a high level of sensitivity. They also suggest that the sensitivity increases in combination with the detection of CK7 mRNA.

Xi and colleagues found that CK-19 had a sensitivity of 100% in detecting tumor in their 21 patients with histologically positive NSCLC nodes. But it was also associated with a low specificity because of the potential amplification of its two known pseudogenes [32]. Bostick and coworkers [27] found that CK-19 mRNA was present in 100% of their breast tumor samples. Unfortunately, they also detected CK-19 mRNA expression in 77% of negative control patients' blood cells and in 100% of their normal lymph nodes. They concluded that the presence of CK-19 in these benign locations diminishes its reliability as a marker for nodal metastasis. This group studied CK-19 with four other markers, namely CEA, GA733.2, MUC1, and CK20. Only CK20 was found to be a reliable marker as it was not detected in any of the blood cells from the healthy donors and none of their normal axillary lymph nodes expressed it. CK20 mRNA detection has yet to be studied in the lymph nodes of NSCLC patients. CK-19 mRNA detection by RT-PCR again has high sensitivity but the existence of pseudogenes makes it difficult to develop a cDNA-specific assay and thus the clinical usefulness of CK19 is diminished [27].

Lung-specific X protein

Lung-specific X protein (Lunx) mRNA and its association with tumor in mediastinal lymph nodes have been studied recently as well. Iwao and colleagues [34] isolated Lunx and localized the gene to chromosome 20. Their study reports the use of RT-PCR for the detection of the mRNA and found it in 84% of their 31 NSCLC tumors and in 0% of their 16 normal lymph nodes. They also detected the mRNA in 80% of their 20 histologically positive lymph nodes. They detected Lunx mRNA in 25% of their histologically negative lymph nodes. Guang-ying and colleagues [35] performed RT-PCR to detect Lunx mRNA in the peripheral blood of 26 patients with lung cancer and 44 regional lymph nodes from 25 patients with lung cancer. Lunx mRNA was detected in the blood of 60% of the NSCLC patients. H&E was performed on the regional lymph nodes and 13.6% of them were found to be histologically positive. RT-PCR detected Lunx in 36.4% of the regional lymph nodes. There was no detection of Lunx mRNA in the blood samples or the lymph nodes of the noncancerous volunteers.

Wallace and colleagues [28] performed RT-PCR on the mediastinal nodes of 87 NSCLC patients without radiological evidence of metastases. They found that Lunx was overexpressed in 15 (56%) of 27 cytology positive mediastinal lymph nodes. They also used an ROC (Receiver Operator Characteristic) analysis, which in this study analyzed the AUC (area under the curve) in a comparison of Lunx's expression in 17 normal samples (control negatives) versus 27 malignant lymph nodes (control positives). An AUC of 1 corresponds to the marker's detection in all of the control positives and no detection in the control negatives. Lunx's AUC was only 0.715, and is likely attributable to its sensitivity of only 56%. In Xi and colleagues' study [31], Lunx was found to have 61.9% sensitivity for the detection of tumor in 21 histologically positive NSCLC nodes. Unlike many of the other discussed markers, Lunx's sensitivity is not particularly high, so many nodes might be missed leading to high rates of false negativity.

RT-PCR has been shown to have increased sensitivity when compared with the standard histopathologic methods currently in use. Many studies, however, reveal that decreased specificity might be a pitfall. Additional investigations are warranted before RT-PCR is made commonplace in the detection of nodal metastasis in NSCLC.

Sentinel lymph node mapping

Although the various molecular strategies discussed may improve the detection of nodal metastases, routine use in all nodes retrieved from a standard mediastinoscopy or mediastinal lymph node dissection is impractical for pathologists. Sentinel lymph node mapping (SLN) in lung cancer has been evaluated in part to address that issue. SLN mapping is now routinely performed in breast cancer and melanoma, which decreases the performance of unnecessary lymph node dissection in some patients. For lung cancer, however, the strategy behind SLN mapping would be to focus advanced pathologic analysis to one or two lymph node stations [36].

Liptay and colleagues [37] performed intraoperative sentinel lymph node mapping in 45 patients with resectable NSCLC. At the time of surgery, they injected the primary tumor with 2 mCi Tc-99 sulfur colloid in the periphery of the tumor. In this study, 37 (82%) of 45 sentinel nodes (labeled as such if their radioactivity measured greater than three times background) were found; 12 (32%) of the 37 nodes had metastatic disease. Of note, 35 (94%) of the 37 sentinel nodes were classified as true positives with no other metastases found in other regional nodes without simultaneous sentinel node involvement. There were 2 (5%) nodes that were inaccurately labeled as sentinel (the sentinel node was negative but another node was positive). In a follow-up study, Liptay and colleagues [37] reported their results of SLN mapping in 90 patients with NSCLC, with similar results: in 86% of patients, at least one SLN was found, and 88.5% of the SLNs were true positives. The results of these studies indicate that sentinel lymph node mapping may be a useful strategy in lymph node staging for patients with NSCLC. Drawbacks include the necessity to use radioactive isotopes in the operating room and the need to wait for the injected isotope to migrate before lymph node or hilar dissection [38]. In addition, the finding of occult N2 disease is less likely to change patient management than when SLN mapping was conceived, owing to broader indications for adjuvant chemotherapy at this time [5]. SLN mapping has been studied in a multi-institutional study by the CALGB, and results are currently being analyzed.

Molecular biologic assessment of prognosis based on lymph node involvement

While it is well understood that lymph node involvement is the most important determinant of prognosis and treatment for patients with potentially resectable lung cancer, the ability to stratify patients is limited to how lymph nodes are characterized by the staging system: N0–N3, without regard to number of involved nodes or extent of malignant involvement [2]. The International Association for the Study of Lung Cancer (IASLC) staging project has addressed this issue, but the proposals for the revision of the N descriptors in the forthcoming seventh edition of the tumor-node-metastasis (TNM) classification will not reflect a change in how lymph nodes are used in staging.

While the assessment of micrometastatic (occult) lymph node involvement may be important in improving prognostic stratification, the use of molecular techniques to assess prognosis (in addition to simply verifying involvement) may be even more powerful. Using IHC techniques, Brooks and colleagues [39] analyzed molecular markers in histologically positive mediastinal nodal specimens obtained from 59 patients without evidence of distant metastatic disease (N2, stage IIIA) treated with induction navelbine-based chemotherapy and external beam radiation therapy followed by surgery. Multivariable analysis of marker expression associated overexpression of p53 and low expression of hMSH2 with poor treatment response and cancer death. Based on this study, it was suggested that molecular biologic analysis might improve the selection of patients with N2 disease for a particular treatment regimen.

Currently, the use of genomic analysis—which has been demonstrated to improve prognostic stratification in patients with early-stage NSCLC—is being used to assess the prognostic and therapeutic implications of N2 involvement [40]. In addition, the use of genomic signature has successfully been used to guide therapy in patients with stage IV NSCLC, and this strategy will be applied to patients with stage III involvement as well, based on the genomic analysis of N2 lymph nodes [41,42].

Summary

Lymph node involvement is the most important factor affecting the prognosis and treatment of patients with potentially resectable NSCLC. Radiographic imaging is inadequate to ascertain lymph node involvement accurately. Currently, lymph nodes are histologically examined with standard histopathologic techniques, such as H&E staining; however, lymph node micrometastases (occult N2 disease) may be missed, leading to inaccurate staging and suboptimal treatment. More accurate strategies, using molecular biologic techniques, are currently being studied.

IHC using antibodies to cytokeratins improves the sensitivity of lymph node assessment. Other techniques, such as RT-PCR, may be superior to IHC, and the detection of various cancer-specific gene transcripts by RT-PCR is being evaluated.

Many transcripts with high sensitivity also demonstrate low specificity, either because of their presence in non-neoplastic tissue or (as is the case of CK-19) because of the existence of associated pseudogenes. At the present time, the most promising molecular detector may be KS1/4, which is infrequently present in noncancerous cells but has a high sensitivity in metastatic nodes. Genomic analysis of lymph nodes, which may be used to improve the detection of micrometastases and to improve risk stratification, is currently being studied. Genomic signatures have the potential to guide therapeutic decision making, as well.

References

[1] Jemal A, Siegel R, Ward E, et al. Cancer statistics, 2008. CA Cancer J Clin 2008;58:71–96.

[2] Mountain CF. Revisions in the international system for staging lung cancer. Chest 1997;111:1710–7.

[3] Rusch VW, Crowley J, Giroux DJ, et al. The IASLC lung cancer staging project: proposals for the revision of the N descriptors in the forthcoming seventh edition of the TNM classification of malignant tumours. J Thorac Oncol 2007;2:603–12.

[4] Goldstraw P, Crowley J, Chansky K, et al. The IASLC lung cancer staging project: proposals for the revision of the TNM stage groupings in the forthcoming (seventh) edition of the TNM classification of malignant tumours. J Thorac Oncol 2007;2: 706–14.

[5] Ettinger DS, Bepler G, Bueno R, et al, National Comprehensive Cancer Network (NCCN). Non-small cell lung cancer clinical practice guidelines in oncology. J Natl Compr Canc Netw 2006;4: 548–82.

[6] Wallace MB, Silvestri GA, Sahai AV, et al. Endoscopic ultrasound-guided fine needle aspiration for staging patients with carcinoma of the lung. Ann Thorac Surg 2001;72:1861–7.

[7] Gonzalez-Stawinski GS, Lemaire A, Merchant FM, et al. A comparative analysis of positron emission tomography and mediastinoscopy in staging patients with non-small cell lung cancer. J Thorac Cardiovasc Surg 2003;126:1900–5.

[8] Graeter TP, Hellwig D, Hoffmann K, et al. Mediastinal lymph node staging in suspected lung cancer: comparison of positron emission tomography with F-18-fluorodeoxyglucose and mediastinoscopy. Ann Thorac Surg 2003;75:231–6.

[9] Reed CE, Harpole DH, Posther KE, et al. Results of the American College of Surgeons Oncology Group Z0050 trial: the utility of positron emission tomography in staging potentially operable non–small cell lung cancer. J Thorac Cardiovasc Surg 2003;126: 1943–51.

[10] Lemaire A, Nikolic I, Petersen T, et al. Nine year single center experience with cervical mediastinoscopy: complications and false negative rate. Ann Thorac Surg 2006;82:1185–90.

[11] de Montpreville VT, Sulmet EM, Nashashibi N. Frozen section diagnosis and surgical biopsy of lymph node tumor and pseudotumors of the mediastinum. Eur J Cardiothorac Surg 1998;13:190–5.

[12] Okubo K, Kato T, Hara A, et al. Imprint cytology for detecting metastasis of lung cancer in mediastinal lymph nodes. Ann Thorac Surg 2004;78:1190–3.

[13] Clarke MR, Landreneau RJ, Borochovits G. Intraoperative imprint cytology for evaluation of mediastinal lymphadenopathy. Ann Thorac Surg 1994;57:1206–10.

[14] D'Amico TA, Massey M, Herndon JE II, et al. A biological risk model for stage I lung cancer: immunohistochemical analysis of 408 patients with the use of ten molecular markers. J Thorac Cardiovasc Surg 1999;117:736–43.

[15] Joshi MB, D'Amico TA, Harpole DH Jr. Molecular biologic substaging of stage I NSCLC through immunohistochemistry performed on formalin-fixed, paraffin-embedded tissue. Methods Mol Med 2003;75:369–88.

[16] Cote RJ, Peterson HF, Chaiwun B, et al. Role of immunohistochemical detection of lymph node metastases in the management of breast cancer. International Breast Cancer Study Group. Lancet 1999;354:896–900.

[17] Passlick B, Izbicki JR, Kubuschok B, et al. Immunohistochemical assessment of individual tumor cells in lymph nodes of patients with non-small-cell lung cancer. J Clin Oncol 1994;12:1827–32.

[18] Vollmer RT, Herndon JE II, D'Cunha J, et al. Immunohistochemical detection of occult lymph node metastases in non-small cell lung cancer: anatomical pathology results from Cancer and Leukemia Group B Trial 9761. Clin Cancer Res 2003;9: 5630–5.

[19] Kubuschok B, Passlick B, Izbicki JR, et al. Disseminated tumor cells in lymph nodes as a determinant for survival in surgically resected non-small cell lung cancer. J Clin Oncol 1999;117:19–24.

[20] Coello MC, Luketich JD, Litle VR, et al. Prognostic significance of micrometastasis in non-small-cell lung cancer. Clin Lung Cancer 2004;4:214–25.

[21] Riquet M, Bagan P, Le Pimpec Barthes F, et al. Completely resected non-small cell lung cancer: reconsidering prognostic value and significance of N2 metastases. Ann Thorac Surg 2007;84:1818–24.

[22] Marchevsky AM, Qiao J, Krajisnik S, et al. The prognostic significance of intranodal isolated tumor cells and micrometastases in patients with non-small cell carcinoma of the lung. J Thorac Cardiovasc Surg 2003;126:551–7.

[23] Goode T, Wen-Zhe H, O'Connor T, et al. Nested RT-PCR. Sensitivity controls are essential to determine the biological significance of detected

mRNA. In: O'Connell J, editor. RT-PCR protocols. Methods in molecular biology, volume 193. Humana Press Inc; 2002. p. 65–79.

[24] Nosotti N, Falleni M, Palleschi A, et al. Quantitative real-time polymerase chain reaction detection of lymph node lung cancer micrometastasis using carcinoembryonic antigen marker. Chest 2005;128: 1539–44.

[25] Mori M, Mimori K, Inoue H, et al. Detection of cancer micrometastases in lymph nodes by reverse transcriptase-polymerase chain reaction. Cancer Res 1995;55:3417–20.

[26] D'Cunha J, Corfits AL, Herndon JE, et al. Molecular staging of lung cancer: real-time polymerase chain reaction estimation of lymph node micrometastatic tumor cell burden in stage I non-small cell lung cancer—preliminary results of cancer and leukemia group B trial 9761. J Thorac Cardiovasc Surg 2002;123:484–91.

[27] Bostick P, Chatterjee S, Chi DD, et al. Limitations of specific reverse-transcriptase polymerase chain reaction markers in the detection of metastases in the lymph nodes and blood of breast cancer patients 16. J Clin Onçol 1998;16:2632–40.

[28] Wallace MB, Block MI, Gillanders W, et al. Accurate molecular detection of non-small cell lung cancer metastases in mediastinal lymph nodes sampled by endoscopic ultrasound-guided needle aspiration. Chest 2005;127:430–7.

[29] Salerno CT, Frizelle S, Niehans GA, et al. Detection of occult micrometastases in non-small cell lung carcinoma by reverse transcriptase-polymerase chain reaction. Chest 1998;113:1526–32.

[30] Saintigny P, Coulon S, Kambouchner M, et al. Real-time RT-PCR detection of CK19, CK7 and MUC1 mRNA for diagnosis of lymph node micrometastases in non-small cell lung carcinoma. Int J Cancer 2005;115:777–82.

[31] Xi L, Coello MC, Litle VR, et al. A combination of molecular markers accurately detects lymph node metastasis in non-small cell lung cancer patients. Clin Cancer Res 2006;12:2484–91.

[32] Mitas M, Cole DJ, Hoover L, et al. Real-time reverse transcription–PCR detects KS1/4 mRNA in mediastinal lymph nodes from patients with non-small cell lung cancer. Clin Chem 2003;49:312–5.

[33] Moll R, Franke W, Schiller D. The catalog of human cytokeratins: patterns of expression in normal epithelia, tumors and cultured cells. Cell 1982;31:11–24.

[34] Iwao K, Watanabe T, Fukiwara Y, et al. Isolation of a novel human lung-specific gene, LUNX, a potential molecular marker for detection of micrometastasis of non-small-cell lung cancer. Int J Cancer 2001;91: 433–7.

[35] Guang-ying Z, De-Lin L, Xu W, et al. Detection of micrometastases of lung cancer by using lunx mRNA specific reverse transcription-polymerase chain reaction. Chinese Journal of Cancer Research 2002;14:54–9.

[36] Liptay MJ, Masters GA, Winchester DJ, et al. Intraoperative radioisotope sentinel lymph node mapping in non–small cell lung cancer. Ann Thorac Surg 2000;70:384–9.

[37] Liptay MJ, Grondin SC, Fry WA, et al. Intraoperative sentinel lymph node mapping non-small cell lung cancer improves detection of micrometastases. J Clin Oncol 2002;20:1984–8.

[38] Liptay MJ. Sentinel node mapping in lung cancer: the holy grail? Ann Thorac Surg 2008;85:S778–9.

[39] Brooks KR, To K, Moore-Joshi M, et al. Measurement of chemotherapy resistance markers in patients with stage III non-small cell lung cancer: a novel approach to patient selection. Ann Thorac Surg 2003;76:187–93.

[40] Potti A, Mukherjee S, Petersen R, et al. A genomic strategy to refine prognosis in early-stage non-small-cell lung cancer. N Engl J Med 2006;355:570–80.

[41] Potti A, Dressman HK, Bild A, et al. Genomic signatures to guide the use of chemotherapeutics. Nat Med 2006;12:1294–300.

[42] Hsu DS, Balakumaran BS, Acharya CR, et al. Pharmacogenomic strategies provide a rational approach to the treatment of cisplatin-resistant patients with advanced cancer. J Clin Oncol 2007;25:4350–7.

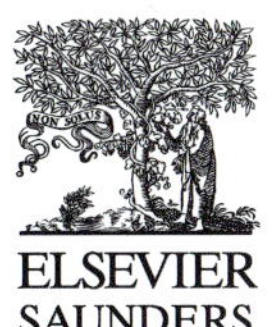
ELSEVIER
SAUNDERS

Thorac Surg Clin 18 (2008) 349–361

THORACIC SURGERY CLINICS

Radiographic Staging of Mediastinal Lymph Nodes in Non–Small Cell Lung Cancer Patients

Shawn S. Groth, MD*, Bryan A. Whitson, MD, PhD, Michael A. Maddaus, MD

University of Minnesota Department of Surgery, Division of General Thoracic and Foregut Surgery, MMC 207, 420 Delaware Street, SE, Minneapolis, MN 55455, USA

Accurate mediastinal lymph node (MLN) staging for non–small cell lung cancer (NSCLC) patients has important therapeutic and prognostic implications [1,2]. Because survival is improved in patients with stage IIIA disease who undergo neoadjuvant chemotherapy followed by surgery, as compared with surgery alone [3–5], the use of sensitive modalities to screen for MLN metastasis is essential. Similarly, patients who are surgical candidates for potentially resectable NSCLC who have completed neoadjuvant therapy for N2 disease require a sensitive and accurate method to restage their mediastinum: those with residual N2 disease found at the time of thoracotomy may not benefit from surgical resection [6,7]. Imaging studies play a vital role in the process of selecting the most appropriate treatment for individual patients.

Chest x-rays

In the initial evaluation of NSCLC patients, posterior-anterior and lateral chest radiographs are valuable. They provide important information regarding underlying cardiopulmonary disease (ie, chronic obstructive pulmonary disease, pulmonary fibrosis, and congestive heart failure) as well as tumor-specific information that contributes to treatment planning (ie, tumor location and size, any obstructive atelectasis, or hilar adenopathy). However, because of their poor sensitivity (less than 50%) [8–10], chest radiographs are an inadequate method to screen for NSCLC MLN metastasis in the absence of obvious, bulky mediastinal adenopathy [8,11]. If the patient is a surgical candidate or needs definitive chemoradiation therapy, additional imaging studies are required.

Computed tomography

Because of its relatively widespread availability and its superior sensitivity, specificity, and diagnostic accuracy, as compared with chest radiographs (Table 1), computed tomography (CT) is the most widely used imaging modality for NSCLC MLN staging in the United States [12]. Despite its advantages over chest radiographs, CT relies on an inaccurate (<70%) method to differentiate benign from malignant MLNs: the size of the MLN. By convention, the criterion of 1 cm is generally used to differentiate potentially malignant MLNs (>1 cm in long-axis diameter) from benign MLNs (<1 cm in long-axis diameter). Using this paradigm, the false-positive rate of CT in the diagnosis of MLN metastasis is 10% to 40% [13,14]; this rate is even higher in patients with central T3 lesions, central adenocarcinomas, or left upper lobe lesions [15]. More importantly, the false-*negative* rate is more than 10% [13,14]. Using CT alone to screen for MLN metastasis would deny patients with false-negative results optimal treatment for their cancer.

Use of alternative MLN anatomic criteria (rather than size) may enhance the sensitivity of CT. In an observational study, Shimoyama and colleagues [16] categorized MLNs as follows: straight or concave MLNs were considered benign and convex MLNs were considered malignant

* Corresponding author.
E-mail address: groth015@umn.edu (S.S. Groth)

1547-4127/08/$ - see front matter
doi:10.1016/j.thorsurg.2008.07.002

Table 1
Radiographic modalities for mediastinal lymph node staging

	References	Sensitivity	Specificity	NPV	PPV	Accuracy
Chest x-ray	[8–10,19]	9% to 47%	78% to 94%	77% to 78%	45% to 80%	68% to 78%
CT	[9,10,19,31, 41–46,49–56, 58,64,120–124]	43% to 87%	59% to 93%	68% to 98%	31% to 84%	59% to 90%
MRI	[8–10,19]	48% to 87%	64% to 91%	—	—	61% to 83%
Standalone PET	[31,40–48,58,64]	50% to 90%	79% to 97%	80% to 99%	42% to 86%	49% to 96%
Visually correlated PET/CT	[40,43,45,64]	67% to 94%	86% to 95%	86%	75%	59% to 88%
PET/CT fusion	[45,46]	78% to 89%	94% to 95%	90% to 94%	88% to 89%	89% to 93%
Integrated PET/CT	[48,64,65,121,124]	60% to 85%	84% to 94%	85% to 99%	49% to 60%	78% to 96%

Sensitivity = true-positives/(true-positives + false-negatives); Specificity = true-negatives/(true-negatives + false-positives); Negative predictive value = true-negatives/(true-negatives + false-negatives); Positive predictive value = true-positives/(true-positives + false-positives); Accuracy = (true-positives + true-negatives)/(true-positives + true-negatives + false-positives + false-negatives).

Abbreviations: CT, computed tomography; FDG, fluorodeoxyglucose; MRI, magnetic resonance imaging; NPV, negative predictive value; PET, positron emission tomography; PPV, positive predictive value; –, no data available.

(regardless of size). Using these criteria, the sensitivity (87.3%), specificity (88.3%), and accuracy (88.1%) of CT for assessing MLNs improved. Additional studies are needed to validate these criteria for malignancy.

Magnetic resonance imaging

As compared with CT, magnetic resonance imaging (MRI) has two distinct advantages: (1) multiplanar imaging (another means of evaluating MLNs that are difficult to assess on axial images) and (2) an enhanced ability to distinguish blood vessels from MLNs, especially in cases where CT is equivocal [17]. In particular, MRI may be more sensitive than CT for evaluating MLNs within the hilum or aortopulmonary window, given its enhanced capacity to distinguish nodal tissue from blood vessels.

Despite its potential advantages, MRI has several disadvantages. Like CT, MRI relies on imprecise anatomic criteria (principally diameter) to diagnose MLN metastasis. MRI also has several distinct disadvantages as compared with CT: (1) less sensitivity for detecting calcification (an indicator of benign disease), (2) inferior spatial resolution (as a result, a group of discrete adjacent normal-sized MLNs may occasionally blur together on MRI and appear as a single large nodal mass, resulting in an erroneous diagnosis of metastasis), (3) longer acquisition time, and (4) higher costs [17].

In part because of those disadvantages, MRI's sensitivity, specificity, and accuracy are similar to those of CT for detecting MLN metastasis (see Table 1) [9,10,18–20]. Several prospective studies comparing the efficacy of CT versus MRI for assessing MLNs for metastasis demonstrated no significant difference in their sensitivity or accuracy [9,10,19]. The use of standard anatomic MRI for staging the mediastinum is currently limited to patients whose CT findings are indeterminate or where the patient has a contrast allergy [21].

Emerging MRI techniques—short-time inversion-recovery turbo spin-echo MRI [22], high (3.0-T) magnetic field MRI [23], and the use of lymphophilic supraparamagnetic agents [17,24,25] —may offer an enhanced capacity to detect MLN metastasis in the future. Until then, CT is preferable to MRI for most NSCLC patients.

Because of the limitations of CT and MRI in staging the mediastinum, functional imaging has emerged as a valuable adjunct.

Positron emission tomography

Radiotracers

Positron emission tomography (PET) involves the use of a systemically administered radiotracer that undergoes decay by emitting positrons (the antiparticle of electrons). The positrons collide with surrounding electrons, thereby creating two photons that move in opposite directions. The photons are ultimately detected and processed by the PET scanner.

The mostly common PET radiotracer is 18-fluorodeoxyglucose (^{18}FDG), a glucose analog that is taken up by cells catabolizing glucose (via glycolysis) and is phosphorylated by the first enzyme in the glycolytic pathway (hexokinase). Because the hydroxyl group on the second carbon of glucose (which is required for further glucose metabolism) is replaced with ^{18}F to synthesize ^{18}FDG, phosphorylated ^{18}FDG cannot be metabolized by the next enzyme in the glycolytic pathway (glucose-6-phosphate isomerase). Furthermore, the negative charge on phosphorylated ^{18}FDG prevents it from leaving the cell. As a result, phosphorylated ^{18}FDG is sequestered inside of the cells that absorbed it until it undergoes radioactive decay; ^{18}FDG is then metabolized by continuing through the glycolytic pathway. Cells with a higher metabolic rate (ie, cancer cells) will take up (and sequester) more ^{18}FDG (and therefore emit more positrons) than cells with a lower metabolic rate.

Although FDG is the most widely used PET metabolite, ^{11}C-choline is emerging as a potential superior alternative. Choline is an organic compound that is a critical component of cellular membranes, of cholinergic neurotransmitters, and of biosynthesis pathways. It is taken up by cells via a transmembrane transport protein. Once inside the cell, choline is ultimately metabolized into phosphatidylcholine, which is then integrated into the extracellular membrane. The activity of choline transmembrane transporters, the metabolism of choline via choline kinase, and the rate of cell membrane synthesis are all increased in tumor cells; accordingly, increased ^{11}C-choline activity indicates tumor proliferation [26]. In a prospective comparative study of 29 patients who underwent ^{18}FDG-PET as well as ^{11}C-choline-PET followed by surgical resection and MLN dissection, ^{11}C-choline-PET provided greater sensitivity (100%) than ^{18}FDG-PET (75%) [27]. Additional trials are needed to validate its use.

Maximum standardized uptake value

The amount of radiotracer uptake can be assessed qualitatively (relative to the amount of background radiotracer uptake) or quantitatively. The most widely used quantitative measure of positron emission (the surrogate for metabolic activity) is the standardized uptake value (SUV), which is defined by the following formula:

$$\mathrm{SUV} = \frac{\text{Activity at a pixel within a region of interest } (\mu\text{Ci/mL})}{(\text{Injected dose } [\mu\text{Ci}]/\text{Body weight } [\text{kg}])}$$

The SUV for a region of interest is most commonly reported as the maximum SUV (maxSUV), which is defined by the pixel within a region of interest on the PET scan that exhibits the greatest SUV.

The ideal cutoff for the maxSUV (above which the lesion is deemed to be malignant) has been debated. Traditionally, clinicians and radiologists have designated a maxSUV of 2.5 as the upper limit of normal [28,29]. In a recent retrospective study of 95 NSCLC patients, receiver operating characteristics (ROC) curve analyses (which determine the cutoff point that maximizes the sensitivity and specificity of a particular test) indicated that the optimal SUV cutoff was 2.5 (which was associated with a sensitivity of 89% and a specificity of 84%), providing additional evidence for this cutoff [30].

In an attempt to improve the sensitivity and accuracy of PET, several researchers have challenged the dogma of using a maxSUV of 2.5 to distinguish benign from malignant MLNs, advocating a higher normal limit for the SUV (eg, 4.5 [31] and 5.3 [32]). In their prospective, single-institution study, Bryant and colleagues [32] compared the PET/CT results of 397 NSCLC patients (143 of whom had pathologically proven N2 disease) with their pathologic stage. Using ROC analyses, they demonstrated that a maxSUV of 5.3 optimized the sensitivity (91%), specificity (88%), and accuracy (92%) of PET; these results were superior to those when a cutoff of 2.5 was used. Their results are intriguing, but until more data are available supporting a higher maximum SUV cut-off, 2.5 should be used.

It is difficult to make precise comparisons between studies because of differences in imaging protocols (eg, the dose, rate of administration, and timing of ^{18}FDG), in PET scanner makes and models, and in the basis for analyses (per patients or per MLN). PET-positivity criteria also vary. Some institutions analyze their data qualitatively, others quantitatively (with various cutoffs for maxSUV).

In attempts to facilitate data comparison among institutions, investigators have explored a variety of methods to normalize the maxSUV.

One such method is to use the ratio of the maxSUV of an MLN of interest to the maxSUV of the primary tumor, thereby negating differences in PET image acquisition protocols and scanners among institutions. Using ROC analyses, Cerfolio and Bryant [33] determined that a cutoff of 0.56 maximized the sensitivity (94%) of this ratio (which they called the PET predictive ratio). Their ratio idea is interesting, but additional studies from other institutions are needed to corroborate this method of analysis.

In addition to providing diagnostic information, the maxSUV provides prognostic information as well. Although not specifically referring to MLNs, multiple studies have demonstrated that a maxSUV above a certain cutoff (5 [34,35], 7 [36], or 10 [37–39]) in NSCLC patients is associated with significantly worse survival.

Positron emission tomography systems

PET may be performed as a dedicated (standalone) imaging study or, in combinations, can be coupled with CT.

Standalone positron emission tomography

In one prospective, single-institution study, 102 patients with potentially resectable NSCLC underwent clinical staging with PET and CT, followed by histologic assessment of the mediastinum with mediastinoscopy and/or lymphadenectomy. For those 102 patients, PET (qualitatively assessed) was associated with superior sensitivity (91% PET versus 75% CT) and accuracy (87% PET versus 69% CT) [40]. Multiple other comparative studies that used pathologic confirmation as the gold standard demonstrated that standalone PET has superior sensitivity and diagnostic accuracy, as compared with CT [31,40–57] (see Table 1). The superiority of PET over CT has also been corroborated by several meta-analyses [58–62].

Again, a limitation of CT is that it relies on size criteria to distinguish benign (< 1 cm in long-axis diameter) and malignant (> 1 cm in long-axis diameter) MLNs. One prospective study of 54 patients with suspected or biopsy-proven NSCLC compared the sensitivity, specificity, and accuracy of PET with CT; it found that PET was associated with superior diagnostic efficacy for small (< 1 cm), intermediate (1 to 3 cm), and large (> 3 cm) MLNs, confirming that functional imaging (with PET) is superior to the use of anatomic criteria to screen for MLN metastases (with CT) [31].

Visually correlated positron emission tomography/computed tomography

To amalgamate the advantages of the two techniques, thereby improving their sensitivity and diagnostic accuracy, CT and PET can be visually compared and contrasted. In a study of 33 patients with suspected NSCLC, Fritscher-Ravens and colleagues [43] found that the combination of PET and CT, as compared with standalone PET, was associated with improved sensitivity (81% PET/CT versus 73% PET), specificity (94% PET/CT versus 83% PET), and accuracy (88% PET/CT versus 79% PET); however, their statistical analysis did not allow for a formal comparison of the two techniques.

Visually correlated PET/CT studies require the radiologist to perform a side-by-side comparison of the PET and CT scans. Side-by-side comparison fosters inconsistent interpretation, which can be especially misleading if the studies were performed on different dates [63]. As a result, the precise location of a lesion can be difficult to ascertain [64].

Positron emission tomography/computed tomography fusion

Because of these limitations with visually correlating PET and CT, PET/CT fusion and integrated PET/CT scans have been valuable advances in radiology. To create PET/CT fusion images, a software program creates three-dimensional models of the PET scan and the CT scan, and then uses an algorithm to create overlay images. Like visually correlated PET/CT, PET/CT fusion has improved efficacy as a method to screen for MLN metastasis, as compared with either PET or CT alone. One study of 28 NSCLC patients compared the efficacy of PET alone, CT alone, visually correlated PET/CT, and PET/CT fusion for clinically staging the mediastinum. It found that PET/CT fusion was associated with improved sensitivity (78%), specificity (95%), negative predictive value (88%), and accuracy (89%) [45].

PET/CT fusion has several technical limitations. In particular, the PET and CT scans that are combined for PET/CT fusion may be obtained on different dates, with different scanners, and with different protocols (for breathing), resulting in image misregistration. A significant limitation of PET/CT fusion, misregistration often precludes completion of the fusion process. One small study (25 patients) found that software fusion was unsuccessful for 32% of patients [48].

Integrated positron emission tomography/computed tomography

Integrated (hybrid) images can be obtained from a combined PET/CT scanner. With this technique, 2 images are obtained (one from PET and one from CT) and then merged to create a single image [63]. Because PET and CT images are obtained in the same setting, this technique overcomes the limitations of fusion and results in significantly better co-registration ($P < .05$) [48].

Several series have demonstrated the superiority of integrated PET/CT over standalone PET. One prospective, investigator-blinded study of 129 NSCLC patients found that integrated PET/CT had superior sensitivity (64%), as compared with standalone PET (62%); the accuracy of integrated PET/CT (96%) was also significantly better than standalone PET (93%) [65].

In addition to its enhanced efficacy for nodal staging, as compared with standalone PET [46,48,64], integrated PET/CT is also superior to visually correlated PET/CT. One prospective study focused on 37 patients (of a total of 50 in the study) with biopsy-proven or suspected NSCLC who underwent histologic evaluation of their MLNs: integrated PET/CT demonstrated superior diagnostic accuracy, as compared with visually correlated PET/CT ($P = .021$) [64].

Because of the consistently proven benefits of the combination of CT and PET, the current National Comprehensive Cancer Network (NCCN) Clinical Practice Guidelines in Oncology [66] state that both CT and PET should be part of the initial and pretreatment evaluations of NSCLC patients. If integrated or fusion scanning is not available, PET and CT should be performed sequentially and then visually correlated.

Restaging

Surgical candidates for potentially resectable NSCLC who have completed neoadjuvant therapy for N2 disease require a sensitive and accurate method to restage their mediastinum. Patients with residual N2 disease found at the time of thoracotomy may not benefit from surgical resection [6,7]. The current gold standard for restaging the mediastinum is repeat mediastinoscopy. A time-tested technique, repeat mediastinoscopy is technically more challenging than initial mediastinoscopy (because of scarring from the initial procedure). Furthermore, repeat mediastinoscopy is also associated with lower sensitivity (29% to 73%, repeat, versus 86% to 93%, initial) and diagnostic accuracy (60% to 85%, repeat, versus 93% to 96%, initial) [19,67–75]. Consequently, less invasive modalities for restaging the mediastinum, such as PET and PET/CT, have been explored.

Restaging the mediastinum with standalone PET is associated with a sensitivity of only 20% to 67% [76–81]. As a result, standalone PET is not a reliable screening test for clearance of mediastinal disease after induction therapy and should not be the sole imaging modality in clinical decision making. Basing treatment decisions on standalone PET would "clear" a significant number of patients (>30%) of their mediastinal disease who, in fact, still have it. Most of these "cleared" patients would, unfortunately, proceed to an operation that would likely confer no survival benefit [6,7].

The sensitivity and diagnostic accuracy of integrated PET/CT are lower for restaging than for initial staging of the mediastinum, yet it has shown some promise as a noninvasive restaging modality. Based on a single institution's experience, it appears that repeat integrated PET/CT is best performed 1 month after the last dose of radiation [82].

Two recent prospective studies have demonstrated that integrated PET/CT is associated with a sensitivity of 62% [83] to 77% [69] and with a diagnostic accuracy of 79% [83] to 83% [69]. Integrated PET/CT is especially valuable for biopsy-proven N2 disease: the change in the maxSUV between the preinduction PET/CT and the postinduction PET/CT correlates with the pathologic response [84]. If the maxSUV of an MLN decreases by more than 50%, there is a high likelihood that the MLN has been rendered free of metastatic disease [83]. Furthermore, if the maxSUV decreases by more than 75%, there is a high likelihood that the patient is a complete responder [83].

Limitations of positron emission tomography

An appreciation of the potential limitations of PET (including the causes of false-positive and false-negative results) is imperative for accurate interpretation of PET or PET/CT findings. One general cause of false-positive results (increased PET signal within a non-neoplastic process) occurs in settings of increased glucose metabolism; a common cause is a benign inflammatory process, which exhibits PET-positivity owing to increased glycolytic activity within leukocytes that have accumulated within the inflammatory focus. Thus, chronic inflammatory processes (eg, sarcoidosis and amyloidosis), acute infections (eg, pneumonias), and residual inflammation after local treatment effects (eg, after surgery, chemotherapy, or radiation) may appear PET-positive and should be part of the differential diagnosis when examining PET results [45,85–87].

Adipose tissue, which has low ^{18}FDG uptake, may also affect SUV results. Therefore, PET-positive lesions within a region of high adipose tissue content will have a seemingly higher SUV relative to their surroundings. Consequently, the apparent SUV of lesions in patients with a higher percentage of body fat will be higher than in non-obese patients [63,88].

Other potential causes of false-positive results include pulmonary emboli and pulmonary infarctions [63], atherosclerotic plaques (because of increased glycolytic activity within the leukocytes that migrated into the plaque) [89,90], and brown fat [63]. Brown fat is thermogenic adipose tissue that contains a relatively high number of mitochondria (and therefore undergoes glycolysis at a higher rate, as compared with other [white] adipose tissue) [63]. The key diagnostic feature of brown fat is that it is usually bilateral and symmetric. Of note, the amount of brown fat is influenced by cold exposure (which *increases* the amount present) and β-blocker use (which *decreases* the amount present).

Potential causes of false-*negative* results should also be considered when interpreting PET and PET/CT findings. Tobacco use can have a significant impact on PET results. As compared with nonsmokers, smokers are more likely to have falsely lowered maxSUV results (and therefore are more likely to have false-negative findings), given their higher background of intrathoraic ^{18}FDG uptake [91]. Because the maxSUV is determined by identifying the pixel on the PET image that has the highest uptake value within a region of interest, the pixel that defines the maxSUV will appear less ^{18}FDG-avid relative to its surroundings when the background uptake is high, as compared with an ^{18}FDG-avid pixel within a region with a lower background of uptake.

The patient's glucose levels and exogenous insulin use can have a profound impact on the distribution of ^{18}FDG, and, consequently, can have a significant impact on PET findings. Glucose competitively displaces ^{18}FDG (via Michaelis-Mentin kinetics) from glucose transporters, preventing ^{18}FDG for uptake into cells [92]. Therefore, hyperglycemia could lead to false-negative findings.

Several authors have proposed methods to adjust for glucose levels at the time of the PET image acquisition. Rather than using the SUV (which is influenced by glucose levels) to describe the results, PET data can be used to determine the metabolic rate of glucose consumption (MR_{glu}) within a region of interest (which is *not* influenced by glucose levels). The commonly accepted standard for measuring MR_{glu} is nonlinear regression. However, this technique is complex and highly sensitive to imaging noise, which is especially problematic when the region of interest has a low MR_{glu} (ie, after induction therapy) [93].

In an attempt to circumvent these limitations, other authors have used Patlak's [94] model of FDG metabolism and have demonstrated a high correlation with nonlinear regression [95]. Still, Patlak's model requires complex graphical analysis that can be difficult to incorporate into a nonresearch setting. Furthermore, a recent study of NSCLC patients undergoing repeat PET after induction therapy demonstrated a high correlation between Patlak's methodology and SUV (corrected for body-surface area and serum glucose level) [93]. Thus, SUV (corrected for body-surface area and serum glucose level) provides a less complicated, yet equally accurate method to quantify PET findings. Other authors have shown that adjusting for glucose level improves the sensitivity of SUV measurements [88,96].

Lee and colleagues [96] examined the utility of the product of the SUV and serum glucose in a study of 70 NSCLC patients. By using ROC analyses to choose the glucose-maxSUV product (290.4) that optimized the sensitivity of PET, the sensitivity (76.2%) was significantly improved ($P < .05$), as compared with the sensitivity of the unadjusted maxSUV (47.6%). Further studies are needed to validate these modalities to adjust for glycemic levels.

Despite the paucity of data in the literature on the effects of hyperglycemia on PET findings in NSCLC patients, chronic hyperglycemia (eg, diabetes mellitus) appears to have a less profound impact than acute hyperglycemia. In a retrospective review comparing ^{18}FDG uptake in the primary tumors of 40 diabetic and 145 nondiabetic NSCLC patients, Gorenberg and colleagues [97] noted no significant difference

($P = .70$). In contrast, acute hyperglycemia can have a profound impact on ^{18}FDG uptake. In a study of 15 NSCLC patients whose PET scans were obtained before and after infusion of 20% glucose (to promote acute hyperglycemia), ^{18}FDG uptake significantly decreased ($P < .001$) after glucose infusion, suggesting that acute hyperglycemia can have profound effects on PET findings [98]. To our knowledge, no studies in the literature have specifically addressed MLN ^{18}FDG uptake in patients with diabetes and in patients with acute hyperglycemia. More studies are needed. Until then, PET findings should be interpreted with caution in such patients.

Like glucose levels, insulin levels can also affect SUV determination by influencing the amount of ^{18}FDG available for uptake by cancer cells. Analogous to its effect on glucose, insulin promotes ^{18}FDG uptake into adipose tissue and skeletal muscle, thereby reducing the amount of ^{18}FDG available for uptake by cancer cells [63].

SUV determination can be affected by several MLN anatomic variables that must be kept in mind when interpreting ^{18}FDG-PET scans. For instance, if the MLN of interest is less than twice the spatial resolution of the scanner, partial volume averaging can result in artifactual SUV reduction (a false-negative finding) [63]. The location of the MLN is also important. On average, the maxSUV for MLN metastases is lower for MLNs in the posterior mediastinum (American Thoracic Society [ATS] stations 5, 7, 8, and 9) [99] than in the anterior mediastinum (ATS stations 2, 4, and 6); the reason may be a higher prevalence of brown fat, resulting in higher background uptake (and thus lower maxSUVs) [100]. Consequently, PET has better sensitivity in detecting metastases in the anterior mediastinum (80% to 99%) than in the posterior mediastinum (29% to 88%) [42].

Tumor histologic findings affect the probability of false-negative findings. In particular, MLN metastases from bronchioalveolar carcinomas (BACs) are associated with lower ^{18}FDG uptake as compared with other NSCLC histologic findings, presumably because of the slower rate of proliferation of BACs [63]. Thus, the probability of false-negative findings is higher with BACs, as compared with other NSCLC histologic findings. When PET-positive MLNs have an SUV of 2.5 or higher, only 50% to 60% of BACs are PET-positive, as compared with 85% of other histologic findings [101]. Also, ^{18}FDG avidity appears to differ between BAC subtypes: mixed BACs are more likely to be PET-positive, as compared with pure BACs [102].

Because of these limitations of PET, histologic confirmation of PET findings is required.

Perhaps in the future, as imaging technology improves, we will be able to be more selective in deciding which NSCLC patients need MLN biopsies.

Histologic assessment

Clinical staging with the currently available imaging studies when used alone (ie, CT, MRI, and PET) or in combination (ie, PET/CT) is not enough to base treatment decisions on. Integrated PET/CT scans are the most sensitive and accurate radiographic means of screening for MLN metastases [45,48,65], yet false-positive and false-negative findings are not uncommon. Some authors have argued that pathologic evaluation of MLNs (ie, with mediastinoscopy) before tumor resection is unnecessary if the PET/CT findings are negative for MLN metastases [103,104].

The incidence of occult N2 disease is relatively high (23.5%) in patients with clinical stage N1 disease (by PET/CT) but low (<3%) in patients with clinical stage N0 disease [104,105]. Even patients with slightly enlarged (10 to 15 mm) MLNs that are PET-negative have a post-PET probability for N2 disease of only 5% [62]. Some authors have argued that mediastinoscopy can be avoided in such patients (ie, those with PET-negative MLNs $\leq$ 15 mm) [62,104,105] before tumor resection and lymphadenectomy. Furthermore, most occult N2 disease arises in the posterior mediastinum, which is not readily accessible by mediastinoscopy [106]. Endobronchial ultrasound-guided fine-needle aspiration (EBUS-FNA) and endoscopic ultrasound-guided fine-needle aspiration (EUS-FNA) have emerged as safe, sensitive, and accurate methods for staging the mediastinum in NSCLC patients [107–110]. Using the combination of these two techniques, near-complete mediastinal staging can be achieved, with excellent sensitivity (92% to 99%, EBUS-FNA alone [107,109,111]; 69% to 95%, EUS-FNA alone [112–114]; 93%, EBUS-FNA and EUS-FNA together [113]) with low morbidity and without a skin incision. Therefore, we advocate performing histologic MLN assessment for all patients with NSCLC, regardless of their PET/CT findings.

Table 2
Histologic assessment methods for mediastinal lymph nodes

Station	Mediastinoscopy	TEMLA [125]	Chamberlain procedure [126]	TBNA-FNA [127]	EBUS-FNA [127]	EUS-FNA [128]	VATS	Thoracotomy
2R	•	•	—	•	•	—	•	•
2L	•	•	—	•	•	—	•	•
3	—	•[b]	—	•	•	•	•	•
4R	•	•	—	•	•	—	•	•
4L	•[a]	•[a]	—	•	•	•	•	•
5	—	•	•	—	—	—	•	•
6	—	•	•	—	—	—	•	•
7	•	•	—	•	•	•	•	•
8	—	•	—	—	—	•	•	•
9	—	—	—	—	—	•	•	•
10R	—	—	—	—	•	—	•	•
10L	—	—	—	—	•	—	•	•
11R	—	—	—	—	•	—	•	•
11L	—	—	—	—	•	—	•	•

Bullets indicate that lymph nodes at a particular station can be accessed by a particular biopsy technique. Dashes indicate that the lymph node station cannot be biopsied by that technique.

Abbreviations: EBUS, endobronchial ultrasound; EUS, endoscopic ultrasound; FNA, fine-needle aspiration; TBNA, transbronchial needle aspiration; TEMLA, transcervical extended mediastinal lymphadenectomy; VATS, video-assisted thoracoscopic surgery.

[a] Only proximal MLN are accessible from this station.

[b] Only anterior MLN are accessible from this station.

Knowledge of the ATS MLN stations and of the anatomic limitations of the available methods of obtaining MLN tissue (Table 2) is essential for developing and implementing an effective diagnostic algorithm. In evaluating NSCLC patients, clinicians must consider both the anatomic location of the MLN in question and the expertise of their particular institution. Regardless of the method used for pretreatment staging of the mediastinum, a complete MLN dissection is required for all patients at the time of definitive resection to provide accurate staging [115–118]. A thorough analysis of the accuracy and diagnostic yield of the methods listed in Table 2 is beyond the scope of this review, but has been recently published elsewhere [119].

Summary

In conclusion, accurate pretreatment staging of NSCLC patients is essential so that they undergo the most appropriate treatment. Imaging studies play an integral part in clinical staging. The preferred imaging method for staging the mediastinum is PET/CT, preferably integrated. Until the sensitivity and accuracy of imaging studies are equivalent to the available MLN biopsy techniques, all candidates for definitive therapy require histologic assessment of the mediastinum.

Acknowledgments

We are indebted to Mary Knatterud, PhD, for her invaluable editorial assistance.

References

[1] Mountain CF. Revisions in the International System for staging lung cancer. Chest 1997;111(6):1710–7.

[2] Naruke T, Goya T, Tsuchiya R, et al. Prognosis and survival in resected lung carcinoma based on the new international staging system. J Thorac Cardiovasc Surg 1988;96(3):440–7.

[3] Rusch VW, Albain KS, Crowley JJ, et al. Surgical resection of stage IIIA and stage IIIB non-small-cell lung cancer after concurrent induction chemoradiotherapy. A Southwest Oncology Group trial. J Thorac Cardiovasc Surg 1993;105(1):97–104 [discussion: 104–6].

[4] Rosell R, Gomez-Codina J, Camps C, et al. A randomized trial comparing preoperative chemotherapy plus surgery with surgery alone in patients with non-small-cell lung cancer. N Engl J Med 1994;330(3):153–8.

[5] Roth JA, Fossella F, Komaki R, et al. A randomized trial comparing perioperative chemotherapy and surgery with surgery alone in resectable stage IIIA non-small-cell lung cancer. J Natl Cancer Inst 1994;86(9):673–80.

[6] Bueno R, Richards WG, Swanson SJ, et al. Nodal stage after induction therapy for stage IIIA lung

cancer determines patient survival. Ann Thorac Surg 2000;70(6):1826–31.
[7] Voltolini L, Luzzi L, Ghiribelli C, et al. Results of induction chemotherapy followed by surgical resection in patients with stage IIIA (N2) non-small cell lung cancer: the importance of the nodal downstaging after chemotherapy. Eur J Cardiothorac Surg 2001;20(6):1106–12.
[8] Faling LJ, Pugatch RD, Jung-Legg Y, et al. Computed tomographic scanning of the mediastinum in the staging of bronchogenic carcinoma. Am Rev Respir Dis 1981;124(6):690–5.
[9] Martini N, Heelan R, Westcott J, et al. Comparative merits of conventional, computed tomographic, and magnetic resonance imaging in assessing mediastinal involvement in surgically confirmed lung carcinoma. J Thorac Cardiovasc Surg 1985;90(5):639–48.
[10] Webb WR, Gatsonis C, Zerhouni EA, et al. CT and MR imaging in staging non-small cell bronchogenic carcinoma: report of the Radiologic Diagnostic Oncology Group. Radiology 1991;178(3):705–13.
[11] Lyn BE, Ayoub AW, Saunders MI, et al. Chest radiography or computed tomography in the assessment of lung cancer prior to radiography. Clin Oncol (R Coll Radiol) 1992;4(3):148–53.
[12] Little AG, Rusch VW, Bonner JA, et al. Patterns of surgical care of lung cancer patients. Ann Thorac Surg 2005;80(6):2051–6.
[13] Eggeling S, Martin T, Bottger J, et al. Invasive staging of non-small cell lung cancer—a prospective study. Eur J Cardiothorac Surg 2002;22(5):679–84.
[14] Kerr KM, Lamb D, Wathen CG, et al. Pathological assessment of mediastinal lymph nodes in lung cancer: implications for non-invasive mediastinal staging. Thorax 1992;47(5):337–41.
[15] Daly BD Jr, Faling LJ, Bite G, et al. Mediastinal lymph node evaluation by computed tomography in lung cancer. An analysis of 345 patients grouped by TNM staging, tumor size, and tumor location. J Thorac Cardiovasc Surg 1987;94(5):664–72.
[16] Shimoyama K, Murata K, Takahashi M, et al. Pulmonary hilar lymph node metastases from lung cancer: evaluation based on morphology at thin-section, incremental, dynamic CT. Radiology 1997;203(1):187–95.
[17] Boiselle PM, Patz EF Jr, Vining DJ, et al. Imaging of mediastinal lymph nodes: CT, MR, and FDG PET. Radiographics 1998;18(5):1061–9.
[18] Quint LE, Francis IR, Wahl RL, et al. Preoperative staging of non-small-cell carcinoma of the lung: imaging methods. AJR Am J Roentgenol 1995;164(6): 1349–59.
[19] Patterson GA, Ginsberg RJ, Poon PY, et al. A prospective evaluation of magnetic resonance imaging, computed tomography, and mediastinoscopy in the preoperative assessment of mediastinal node status in bronchogenic carcinoma. J Thorac Cardiovasc Surg 1987;94(5):679–84.
[20] Webb WR, Sarin M, Zerhouni EA, et al. Interobserver variability in CT and MR staging of lung cancer. J Comput Assist Tomogr 1993;17(6):841–6.
[21] Silvestri GA, Tanoue LT, Margolis ML, et al. The noninvasive staging of non-small cell lung cancer: the guidelines. Chest 2003;123(Suppl 1):147S–56S.
[22] Ohno Y, Hatabu H, Takenaka D, et al. Metastases in mediastinal and hilar lymph nodes in patients with non-small cell lung cancer: quantitative and qualitative assessment with STIR turbo spin-echo MR imaging. Radiology 2004;231(3):872–9.
[23] Kim HY, Yi CA, Lee KS, et al. Nodal metastasis in non-small cell lung cancer: accuracy of 3.0-T MR imaging. Radiology 2008;246(2):596–604.
[24] Vassallo P, Matei C, Heston WD, et al. AMI-227-enhanced MR lymphography: usefulness for differentiating reactive from tumor-bearing lymph nodes. Radiology 1994;193(2):501–6.
[25] Weissleder R, Cheng HC, Bogdanova A, et al. Magnetically labeled cells can be detected by MR imaging. J Magn Reson Imaging 1997;7(1):258–63.
[26] Hara T, Kosaka N, Suzuki T, et al. Uptake rates of 18F-fluorodeoxyglucose and 11C-choline in lung cancer and pulmonary tuberculosis: a positron emission tomography study. Chest 2003;124(3): 893–901.
[27] Hara T, Inagaki K, Kosaka N, et al. Sensitive detection of mediastinal lymph node metastasis of lung cancer with 11C-choline PET. J Nucl Med 2000;41(9):1507–13.
[28] Menda Y, Bushnell DL, Madsen MT, et al. Evaluation of various corrections to the standardized uptake value for diagnosis of pulmonary malignancy. Nucl Med Commun 2001;22(10):1077–81.
[29] Patz EF Jr, Lowe VJ, Hoffman JM, et al. Focal pulmonary abnormalities: evaluation with F-18 fluorodeoxyglucose PET scanning. Radiology 1993; 188(2):487–90.
[30] Hellwig D, Graeter TP, Ukena D, et al. 18F-FDG PET for mediastinal staging of lung cancer: which SUV threshold makes sense? J Nucl Med 2007; 48(11):1761–6.
[31] Gupta NC, Graeber GM, Bishop HA. Comparative efficacy of positron emission tomography with fluorodeoxyglucose in evaluation of small (3 cm) lymph node lesions. Chest 2000;117(3):773–8.
[32] Bryant AS, Cerfolio RJ, Klemm KM, et al. Maximum standard uptake value of mediastinal lymph nodes on integrated FDG-PET-CT predicts pathology in patients with non-small cell lung cancer. Ann Thorac Surg 2006;82(2):417–22 [discussion: 422–3].
[33] Cerfolio RJ, Bryant AS. Ratio of the maximum standardized uptake value on FDG-PET of the mediastinal (N2) lymph nodes to the primary tumor may be a universal predictor of nodal malignancy in patients with nonsmall-cell lung cancer. Ann Thorac Surg 2007;83(5):1826–9 [discussion: 1829–30].

[34] Sasaki R, Komaki R, Macapinlac H, et al. SUV by FDG-PET predicts outcomes of NSCLC. Int J Radiat Oncol Biol Phys 2003;57(Suppl 2):S166.

[35] Higashi K, Ueda Y, Arisaka Y, et al. 18F-FDG uptake as a biologic prognostic factor for recurrence in patients with surgically resected non-small cell lung cancer. J Nucl Med 2002;43(1):39–45.

[36] Vansteenkiste JF, Stroobants SG, Dupont PJ, et al. Prognostic importance of the standardized uptake value on (18)F-fluoro-2-deoxy-glucose-positron emission tomography scan in non-small-cell lung cancer: an analysis of 125 cases. Leuven Lung Cancer Group. J Clin Oncol 1999;17(10):3201–6.

[37] Ahuja V, Coleman RE, Herndon J, et al. The prognostic significance of fluorodeoxyglucose positron emission tomography imaging for patients with nonsmall cell lung carcinoma. Cancer 1998;83(5): 918–24.

[38] Cerfolio RJ, Bryant AS, Ohja B, et al. The maximum standardized uptake values on positron emission tomography of a non-small cell lung cancer predict stage, recurrence, and survival. J Thorac Cardiovasc Surg 2005;130(1):151–9.

[39] Downey RJ, Akhurst T, Gonen M, et al. Preoperative F-18 fluorodeoxyglucose-positron emission tomography maximal standardized uptake value predicts survival after lung cancer resection. J Clin Oncol 2004;22(16):3255–60.

[40] Pieterman RM, van Putten JW, Meuzelaar JJ, et al. Preoperative staging of non-small-cell lung cancer with positron-emission tomography. N Engl J Med 2000;343(4):254–61.

[41] Bury T, Paulus P, Dowlati A, et al. Staging of the mediastinum: value of positron emission tomography imaging in non-small cell lung cancer. Eur Respir J 1996;9(12):2560–4.

[42] Cerfolio RJ, Ojha B, Bryant AS, et al. The role of FDG-PET scan in staging patients with nonsmall cell carcinoma. Ann Thorac Surg 2003;76(3):861–6.

[43] Fritscher-Ravens A, Bohuslavizki KH, Brandt L, et al. Mediastinal lymph node involvement in potentially resectable lung cancer: comparison of CT, positron emission tomography, and endoscopic ultrasonography with and without fine-needle aspiration. Chest 2003;123(2):442–51.

[44] Luketich JD, Friedman DM, Meltzer CC, et al. The role of positron emission tomography in evaluating mediastinal lymph node metastases in non-small-cell lung cancer. Clin Lung Cancer 2001;2(3): 229–33.

[45] Magnani P, Carretta A, Rizzo G, et al. FDG/PET and spiral CT image fusion for medistinal lymph node assessment of non-small cell lung cancer patients. J Cardiovasc Surg (Torino) 1999;40(5): 741–8.

[46] Antoch G, Stattaus J, Nemat AT, et al. Non-small cell lung cancer: dual-modality PET/CT in preoperative staging. Radiology 2003;229(2):526–33.

[47] Vesselle H, Pugsley JM, Vallieres E, et al. The impact of fluorodeoxyglucose F 18 positron-emission tomography on the surgical staging of non-small cell lung cancer. J Thorac Cardiovasc Surg 2002; 124(3):511–9.

[48] Halpern BS, Schiepers C, Weber WA, et al. Presurgical staging of non-small cell lung cancer: positron emission tomography, integrated positron emission tomography/CT, and software image fusion. Chest 2005;128(4):2289–97.

[49] Chin R Jr, Ward R, Keyes JW, et al. Mediastinal staging of non-small-cell lung cancer with positron emission tomography. Am J Respir Crit Care Med 1995;152(6 Pt 1):2090–6.

[50] Guhlmann A, Storck M, Kotzerke J, et al. Lymph node staging in non-small cell lung cancer: evaluation by [18F]FDG positron emission tomography (PET). Thorax 1997;52(5):438–41.

[51] Sasaki M, Ichiya Y, Kuwabara Y, et al. The usefulness of FDG positron emission tomography for the detection of mediastinal lymph node metastases in patients with non-small cell lung cancer: a comparative study with x-ray computed tomography. Eur J Nucl Med 1996;23(7):741–7.

[52] Sazon DA, Santiago SM, Soo Hoo GW, et al. Fluorodeoxyglucose-positron emission tomography in the detection and staging of lung cancer. Am J Respir Crit Care Med 1996;153(1):417–21.

[53] Scott WJ, Gobar LS, Terry JD, et al. Mediastinal lymph node staging of non-small-cell lung cancer: a prospective comparison of computed tomography and positron emission tomography. J Thorac Cardiovasc Surg 1996;111(3):642–8.

[54] Steinert HC, Hauser M, Allemann F, et al. Non-small cell lung cancer: nodal staging with FDG PET versus CT with correlative lymph node mapping and sampling. Radiology 1997;202(2):441–6.

[55] Vansteenkiste JF, Stroobants SG, De Leyn PR, et al. Mediastinal lymph node staging with FDG-PET scan in patients with potentially operable non-small cell lung cancer: a prospective analysis of 50 cases. Leuven Lung Cancer Group. Chest 1997;112(6):1480–6.

[56] Weng E, Tran L, Rege S, et al. Accuracy and clinical impact of mediastinal lymph node staging with FDG-PET imaging in potentially resectable lung cancer. Am J Clin Oncol 2000;23(1):47–52.

[57] Ebihara A, Nomori H, Watanabe K, et al. Characteristics of advantages of positron emission tomography over computed tomography for N-staging in lung cancer patients. Jpn J Clin Oncol 2006;36(11): 694–8.

[58] Birim O, Kappetein AP, Stijnen T, et al. Meta-analysis of positron emission tomographic and computed tomographic imaging in detecting mediastinal lymph node metastases in nonsmall cell lung cancer. Ann Thorac Surg 2005;79(1): 375–82.

[59] Alongi F, Ragusa P, Montemaggi P, et al. Combining independent studies of diagnostic fluorodeoxyglucose positron-emission tomography and computed tomography in mediastinal lymph node staging for non-small cell lung cancer. Tumori 2006;92(4):327–33.

[60] Dwamena BA, Sonnad SS, Angobaldo JO, et al. Metastases from non-small cell lung cancer: mediastinal staging in the 1990s—meta-analytic comparison of PET and CT. Radiology 1999;213(2): 530–6.

[61] Toloza EM, Harpole L, McCrory DC. Noninvasive staging of non-small cell lung cancer: a review of the current evidence. Chest 2003;123(Suppl 1): 137S–46S.

[62] Gould MK, Kuschner WG, Rydzak CE, et al. Test performance of positron emission tomography and computed tomography for mediastinal staging in patients with non-small-cell lung cancer: a meta-analysis. Ann Intern Med 2003;139(11):879–92.

[63] Cerfolio RJ, Bryant AS. The role of integrated positron emission tomography-computerized tomography in evaluating and staging patients with non-small cell lung cancer. Semin Thorac Cardiovasc Surg 2007;19(3):192–200.

[64] Lardinois D, Weder W, Hany TF, et al. Staging of non-small-cell lung cancer with integrated positron-emission tomography and computed tomography. N Engl J Med 2003;348(25):2500–7.

[65] Cerfolio RJ, Ojha B, Bryant AS, et al. The accuracy of integrated PET-CT compared with dedicated PET alone for the staging of patients with nonsmall cell lung cancer. Ann Thorac Surg 2004;78(3): 1017–23 [discussion: 1017–23].

[66] The NCCN non-small cell lung cancer clinical practice guidelines in oncology (version 1.2007) Available at: http://www.nccn.org. Accessed August 25, 2007.

[67] Van Schil P, van der Schoot J, Poniewierski J, et al. Remediastinoscopy after neoadjuvant therapy for non-small cell lung cancer. Lung Cancer 2002; 37(3):281–5.

[68] Mateu-Navarro M, Rami-Porta R, Bastus-Piulats R, et al. Remediastinoscopy after induction chemotherapy in non-small cell lung cancer. Ann Thorac Surg 2000;70(2):391–5.

[69] De Leyn P, Stroobants S, De Wever W, et al. Prospective comparative study of integrated positron emission tomography-computed tomography scan compared with remediastinoscopy in the assessment of residual mediastinal lymph node disease after induction chemotherapy for mediastinoscopy-proven stage IIIA-N2 Non-small-cell lung cancer: a Leuven Lung Cancer Group Study. J Clin Oncol 2006;24(21):3333–9.

[70] Coughlin M, Deslauriers J, Beaulieu M, et al. Role of mediastinoscopy in pretreatment staging of patients with primary lung cancer. Ann Thorac Surg 1985;40(6):556–60.

[71] Cybulsky IJ, Bennett WF. Mediastinoscopy as a routine outpatient procedure. Ann Thorac Surg 1994;58(1):176–8.

[72] Hammoud ZT, Anderson RC, Meyers BF, et al. The current role of mediastinoscopy in the evaluation of thoracic disease. J Thorac Cardiovasc Surg 1999;118(5):894–9.

[73] Lemaire A, Nikolic I, Petersen T, et al. Nine-year single center experience with cervical mediastinoscopy: complications and false negative rate. Ann Thorac Surg 2006;82(4):1185–9 [discussion: 1189–90].

[74] Luke WP, Pearson FG, Todd TR, et al. Prospective evaluation of mediastinoscopy for assessment of carcinoma of the lung. J Thorac Cardiovasc Surg 1986;91(1):53–6.

[75] Pauwels M, Van Schil P, De Backer W, et al. Repeat mediastinoscopy in the staging of lung cancer. Eur J Cardiothorac Surg 1998;14(3):271–3.

[76] Vansteenkiste J, Stroobants S, Hoekstra C, et al. 18Fluoro-2-deoxyglucose positron emission tomography (PET) in the assessment of induction chemotherapy (IC) in stage IIIa-N2 NSCLC: a multi-center prospective study [abstract]. Proc Am Soc Clin Oncol 2001;20(313A):1250.

[77] Akhurst T, Downey RJ, Ginsberg MS, et al. An initial experience with FDG-PET in the imaging of residual disease after induction therapy for lung cancer. Ann Thorac Surg 2002;73(1):259–64 [discussion: 264–6].

[78] Ryu JS, Choi NC, Fischman AJ, et al. FDG-PET in staging and restaging non-small cell lung cancer after neoadjuvant chemoradiotherapy: correlation with histopathology. Lung Cancer 2002;35(2): 179–87.

[79] Cerfolio RJ, Ojha B, Mukherjee S, et al. Positron emission tomography scanning with 2-fluoro-2-deoxy-d-glucose as a predictor of response of neoadjuvant treatment for non-small cell carcinoma. J Thorac Cardiovasc Surg 2003;125(4):938–44.

[80] Port JL, Kent MS, Korst RJ, et al. Positron emission tomography scanning poorly predicts response to preoperative chemotherapy in non-small cell lung cancer. Ann Thorac Surg 2004;77(1):254–9 [discussion: 259].

[81] Hellwig D, Graeter TP, Ukena D, et al. Value of F-18-fluorodeoxyglucose positron emission tomography after induction therapy of locally advanced bronchogenic carcinoma. J Thorac Cardiovasc Surg 2004;128(6):892–9.

[82] Cerfolio RJ, Bryant AS. When is it best to repeat a 2-fluoro-2-deoxy-D-glucose positron emission tomography/computed tomography scan on patients with non-small cell lung cancer who have received neoadjuvant chemoradiotherapy? Ann Thorac Surg 2007;84(4):1092–7.

[83] Cerfolio RJ, Bryant AS, Ojha B. Restaging patients with N2 (stage IIIA) non-small cell lung cancer after neoadjuvant chemoradiotherapy:

a prospective study. J Thorac Cardiovasc Surg 2006;131(6):1229–35.

[84] Cerfolio RJ, Bryant AS, Winokur TS, et al. Repeat FDG-PET after neoadjuvant therapy is a predictor of pathologic response in patients with non-small cell lung cancer. Ann Thorac Surg 2004;78(6): 1903–9 [discussion: 1909].

[85] Belhocine T, De Barsy C, Hustinx R, et al. Usefulness of (18)F-FDG PET in the post-therapy surveillance of endometrial carcinoma. Eur J Nucl Med Mol Imaging 2002;29(9):1132–9.

[86] Ryu SY, Kim MH, Choi SC, et al. Detection of early recurrence with 18F-FDG PET in patients with cervical cancer. J Nucl Med 2003;44(3):347–52.

[87] Yen TC, Lai CH. Positron emission tomography in gynecologic cancer. Semin Nucl Med 2006;36(1): 93–104.

[88] Yeung, Dwc, Yeung, et al. Improving reproducibility of SUV by FDG dose adjusted for body size and serum glucose level. Clin Positron Imaging 2000; 3(4):177.

[89] Rudd JH, Warburton EA, Fryer TD, et al. Imaging atherosclerotic plaque inflammation with [18F]-fluorodeoxyglucose positron emission tomography. Circulation 2002;105(23):2708–11.

[90] Asad S, Aquino SL, Piyavisetpat N, et al. False-positive FDG positron emission tomography uptake in nonmalignant chest abnormalities. AJR Am J Roentgenol 2004;182(4):983–9.

[91] Bryant AS, Cerfolio RJ. The clinical stage of non-small cell lung cancer as assessed by means of fluorodeoxyglucose-positron emission tomographic/computed tomographic scanning is less accurate in cigarette smokers. J Thorac Cardiovasc Surg 2006;132(6):1363–8.

[92] Yamada K, Endo S, Fukuda H, et al. Experimental studies on myocardial glucose metabolism of rats with 18F-2-fluoro-2-deoxy-D-glucose. Eur J Nucl Med 1985;10(7–8):341–5.

[93] Hoekstra CJ, Stroobants SG, Smit EF, et al. Prognostic relevance of response evaluation using [18F]-2-fluoro-2-deoxy-D-glucose positron emission tomography in patients with locally advanced non-small-cell lung cancer. J Clin Oncol 2005; 23(33):8362–70.

[94] Patlak CS, Blasberg RG, Fenstermacher JD. Graphical evaluation of blood-to-brain transfer constants from multiple-time uptake data. J Cereb Blood Flow Metab 1983;3(1):1–7.

[95] Hoekstra CJ, Hoekstra OS, Stroobants SG, et al. Methods to monitor response to chemotherapy in non-small cell lung cancer with 18F-FDG PET. J Nucl Med 2002;43(10):1304–9.

[96] Lee WW, Chung JH, Jang SJ, et al. Consideration of serum glucose levels during malignant mediastinal lymph node detection in non-small-cell lung cancer by FDG-PET. J Surg Oncol 2006;94(7):607–13.

[97] Gorenberg M, Hallett WA, O'Doherty MJ. Does diabetes affect [(18)F]FDG standardised uptake values in lung cancer? Eur J Nucl Med Mol Imaging 2002;29(10):1324–7.

[98] Langen KJ, Braun U, Rota Kops E, et al. The influence of plasma glucose levels on fluorine-18-fluorodeoxyglucose uptake in bronchial carcinomas. J Nucl Med 1993;34(3):355–9.

[99] Mountain CF, Dresler CM. Regional lymph node classification for lung cancer staging. Chest 1997; 111(6):1718–23.

[100] Truong MT, Erasmus JJ, Munden RF, et al. Focal FDG uptake in mediastinal brown fat mimicking malignancy: a potential pitfall resolved on PET/CT. AJR Am J Roentgenol 2004;183(4):1127–32.

[101] Heyneman LE, Patz EF. PET imaging in patients with bronchioloalveolar cell carcinoma. Lung Cancer 2002;38(3):261–6.

[102] Yap CS, Schiepers C, Fishbein MC, et al. FDG-PET imaging in lung cancer: how sensitive is it for bronchioloalveolar carcinoma? Eur J Nucl Med Mol Imaging 2002;29(9):1166–73.

[103] Schimmer C, Neukam K, Elert O. Staging of non-small cell lung cancer: clinical value of positron emission tomography and mediastinoscopy. Interact Cardiovasc Thorac Surg 2006;5(4):418–23.

[104] Meyers BF, Haddad F, Siegel BA, et al. Cost-effectiveness of routine mediastinoscopy in computed tomography- and positron emission tomography-screened patients with stage I lung cancer. J Thorac Cardiovasc Surg 2006;131(4):822–9 [discussion: 8229].

[105] Cerfolio RJ, Bryant AS, Eloubeidi MA. Routine mediastinoscopy and esophageal ultrasound fine-needle aspiration in patients with non-small cell lung cancer who are clinically N2 negative: a prospective study. Chest 2006;130(6):1791–5.

[106] Cerfolio RJ, Bryant AS, Ojha B, et al. Improving the inaccuracies of clinical staging of patients with NSCLC: a prospective trial. Ann Thorac Surg 2005;80(4):1207–13 [discussion: 1213–4].

[107] Herth FJ, Eberhardt R, Vilmann P, et al. Real-time endobronchial ultrasound guided transbronchial needle aspiration for sampling mediastinal lymph nodes. Thorax 2006;61(9):795–8.

[108] Yasufuku K, Chiyo M, Koh E, et al. Endobronchial ultrasound guided transbronchial needle aspiration for staging of lung cancer. Lung Cancer 2005;50(3):347–54.

[109] Vincent BD, El-Bayoumi E, Hoffman B, et al. Real-time endobronchial ultrasound-guided transbronchial lymph node aspiration. Ann Thorac Surg 2008;85(1):224–30.

[110] Herth FJ, Rabe KF, Gasparini S, et al. Transbronchial and transoesophageal (ultrasound-guided) needle aspirations for the analysis of mediastinal lesions. Eur Respir J 2006;28(6):1264–75.

[111] Yasufuku K, Nakajima T, Motoori K, et al. Comparison of endobronchial ultrasound, positron emission tomography, and CT for lymph node staging of lung cancer. Chest 2006;130(3):710–8.

[112] Caddy G, Conron M, Wright G, et al. The accuracy of EUS-FNA in assessing mediastinal lymphadenopathy and staging patients with NSCLC. Eur Respir J 2005;25(3):410–5.

[113] Wallace MB, Pascual JM, Raimondo M, et al. Minimally invasive endoscopic staging of suspected lung cancer. JAMA 2008;299(5):540–6.

[114] Gress FG, Savides TJ, Sandler A, et al. Endoscopic ultrasonography, fine-needle aspiration biopsy guided by endoscopic ultrasonography, and computed tomography in the preoperative staging of non-small-cell lung cancer: a comparison study. Ann Intern Med 1997;127(8 Pt 1):604–12.

[115] Allen MS, Darling GE, Pechet TT, et al. Morbidity and mortality of major pulmonary resections in patients with early-stage lung cancer: initial results of the randomized, prospective ACOSOG Z0030 trial. Ann Thorac Surg 2006;81(3):1013–9.

[116] Doddoli C, Aragon A, Barlesi F, et al. Does the extent of lymph node dissection influence outcome in patients with stage I non-small-cell lung cancer? Eur J Cardiothorac Surg 2005;27(4):680–5.

[117] Gajra A, Newman N, Gamble GP, et al. Effect of number of lymph nodes sampled on outcome in patients with stage I non-small-cell lung cancer. J Clin Oncol 2003;21(6):1029–34.

[118] Keller SM, Adak S, Wagner H, et al. A randomized trial of postoperative adjuvant therapy in patients with completely resected stage II or IIIA non-small-cell lung cancer. Eastern Cooperative Oncology Group. N Engl J Med 2000;343(17):1217–22.

[119] Whitson BA, Groth SS, Maddaus MA. Surgical assessment and intraoperative management of mediastinal lymph nodes in non-small cell lung cancer. Ann Thorac Surg 2007;84(3):1059–65.

[120] Egri G, Meszaros Z, Vass G, et al. How effective is the routine mediastinal block dissection in the surgery of non-small cell lung cancer? Acta Chir Hung 1998;37(1–2):85–93.

[121] Shim SS, Lee KS, Kim BT, et al. Non-small cell lung cancer: prospective comparison of integrated FDG PET/CT and CT alone for preoperative staging. Radiology 2005;236(3):1011–9.

[122] Graeter TP, Hellwig D, Hoffmann K, et al. Mediastinal lymph node staging in suspected lung cancer: comparison of positron emission tomography with F-18-fluorodeoxyglucose and mediastinoscopy. Ann Thorac Surg 2003;75(1):231–5 [discussion: 235–6].

[123] Roberts PF, Follette DM, von Haag D, et al. Factors associated with false-positive staging of lung cancer by positron emission tomography. Ann Thorac Surg 2000;70(4):1154–9 [discussion: 1159–60].

[124] Tournoy KG, Maddens S, Gosselin R, et al. Integrated FDG-PET/CT does not make invasive staging of the intrathoracic lymph nodes in non-small cell lung cancer redundant: a prospective study. Thorax 2007;62(8):696–701.

[125] Kuzdzal J, Zielinski M, Papla B, et al. Transcervical extended mediastinal lymphadenectomy—the new operative technique and early results in lung cancer staging. Eur J Cardiothorac Surg 2005; 27(3):384–90 [discussion: 390].

[126] McNeill TM, Chamberlain JM. Diagnostic anterior mediastinotomy. Ann Thorac Surg 1966;2(4):532–9.

[127] Herth F, Becker HD, Ernst A. Conventional vs endobronchial ultrasound-guided transbronchial needle aspiration: a randomized trial. Chest 2004; 125(1):322–5.

[128] Annema JT, Versteegh MI, Veselic M, et al. Endoscopic ultrasound added to mediastinoscopy for preoperative staging of patients with lung cancer. JAMA 2005;294(8):931–6.

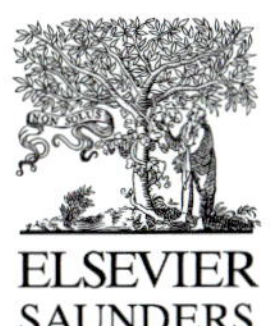

ELSEVIER
SAUNDERS

Thorac Surg Clin 18 (2008) 363–379

THORACIC
SURGERY
CLINICS

Minimally Invasive Staging of N2 Disease: Endobronchial Ultrasound/Transesophageal Endoscopic Ultrasound, Mediastinoscopy, and Thoracoscopy

Paul Schipper, MD, FACS, FACCP*, Matt Schoolfield, MD

Section of General Thoracic Surgery, Division of Cardiothoracic Surgery, Department of Surgery, Mail Code L353, Oregon Health and Sciences University, 3181 SW Sam Jackson Park Road, Portland, OR 97229, USA

The treatments for lung cancer, whether chemotherapy, radiation therapy, or surgery, are toxic. Before embarking on a treatment plan, the clinician and patient would like assurance that the benefits of these treatments in survival and quality of life are worth enduring this toxicity. To assist in choosing appropriate therapy, the lung cancer staging system was developed. A key turning point in the staging system with regards to prognosis and treatment decision-making is the presence or absence of metastatic disease in the N2 lymph nodes. Failure to consider or to evaluate these lymph nodes adequately does not make them any more or less likely to be involved. Such failure can, however, increase the chances of making an error in the treatment. This error can happen in both directions. A patient who has undiscovered positive N2 lymph nodes (a false-negative finding) can be treated with an extensive and invasive surgery with little chance of benefit. Conversely, a patient incorrectly diagnosed as having positive N2 lymph nodes (a false-positive finding) can be denied a chance of curative therapy.

Current treatment for stage IIIA lung cancer is detailed elsewhere in this issue. In brief, a patient who has known disease metastatic to the N2 lymph nodes but no distant disease is treated with multimodality therapy beginning with chemotherapy and radiation therapy and possibly followed by surgery [1–14]. Surgery generally is not an initial treatment for stage IIIA lung cancer. Surgery remains the initial treatment for stage I through stage IIB lung cancer. In some instances, an increased survival advantage is found with postoperative chemotherapy and/or radiation therapy for select stage IB, IIA, and IIB disease. The utility of preoperative chemotherapy and radiation therapy for stage I through stage IIB lung cancer is not known, and trials examining this issue are ongoing.

The gold standard for N2 lymph node evaluation is surgical resection of those lymph nodes at the time of thoracoscopy or thoracotomy. The clinician is left with the dilemma that the best means of evaluating the lymph nodes in question potentially involves much of the toxicity that should be avoided if those lymph nodes are positive. To answer this dilemma, multiple methods of minimally invasive evaluation of the N2 lymph nodes have been developed in hope of providing information similar to that obtained by a lymphadenectomy but with less morbidity. Techniques such as chest CT and positron emission tomography (PET) scan, although involving invasion and subsequent risk to the patient in the form of radiation and intravenous contrast, generally are considered noninvasive. A thoracotomy with lymphadenectomy is considered maximally invasive. Between these extremes are a range of

* Corresponding author.
E-mail address: schippep@ohsu.edu (P. Schipper).

1547-4127/08/$ - see front matter
doi:10.1016/j.thorsurg.2008.08.001

minimally invasive procedures consisting of endobronchial ultrasound (EBUS) and needle biopsy, endoscopic transesophageal ultrasound (EUS) and needle biopsy, cervical mediastinoscopy and biopsy, and thoracoscopy and biopsy.

This article details these four minimally invasive procedures, the lymph nodes they are able to evaluate, the limitations of the procedures, any available additional information the procedures can yield beyond lymph node staging, what is known about the procedures' ability to determine whether there is cancer in the N2 lymph nodes, and most importantly, the potential cost to the patient in answering that question.

What are N2 lymph nodes?

N2 lymph nodes, as defined by the sixth edition of the American Joint Commission on Cancer (AJCC) and Union Internationale Contre le Cancer (UICC) staging manuals, are the ipsilateral mediastinal and/or subcarinal lymph nodes. They are distinguished from N3 nodes, which are contralateral mediastinal, contralateral hilar, or ipsilateral, or contralateral scalene or supraclavicular lymph nodes. They also are distinguished from the N1 nodes, which are the ipsilateral peribronchial, ipsilateral hilar, and ipsilateral intraparenchymal lymph nodes [15,16]. No changes to the N descriptors are proposed for the upcoming seventh editions of the AJCC and UICC cancer staging manuals [17]. Worldwide, two mediastinal lymph node maps are in use. One, developed by Naruke [18], is used primarily in Japan. The other is the Mountain-Dresler modification of the American Thoracic Society map (Figs. 1, 2). The differences between these maps are well defined by Rusch and colleagues [17] and are presented in Table 1. In both, the single-digit lymph node stations define the mediastinal nodes and, depending on the relationship between the primary lung cancer and the node, are either N2 or N3. The only significant difference between these two maps in determining N2 disease is in the subcarinal position. The Naruke map defines the lymphatic material next to the left and right mainstem bronchi as level 10 and therefore N1. The Mountain-Dresler map defines this location as part of level 7 and therefore N2. Knowing which system is being used is important in evaluating the literature, assessing the ability of a modality to reach certain stations, and communicating findings between the physician performing the biopsy and the physician using that information. For

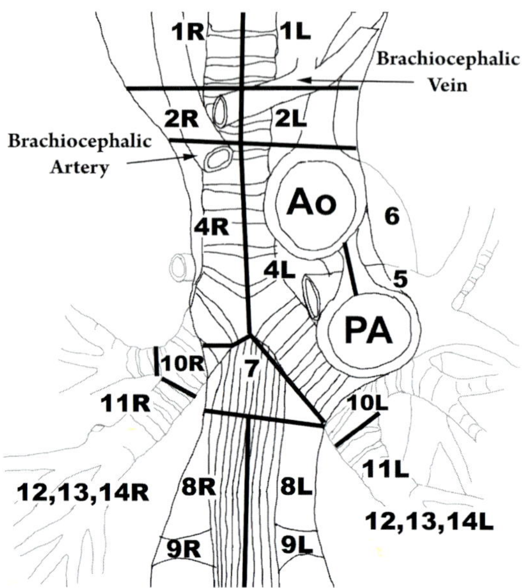

Fig. 1. Mountain-Dressler thoracic lymph node map. anterior-posterior view. AO: aorta, PA: pulmonary artery. (*Data from* Mountain CF. Revisions in the international system for staging lung cancer. Chest 1997;111(6):1710–7.)

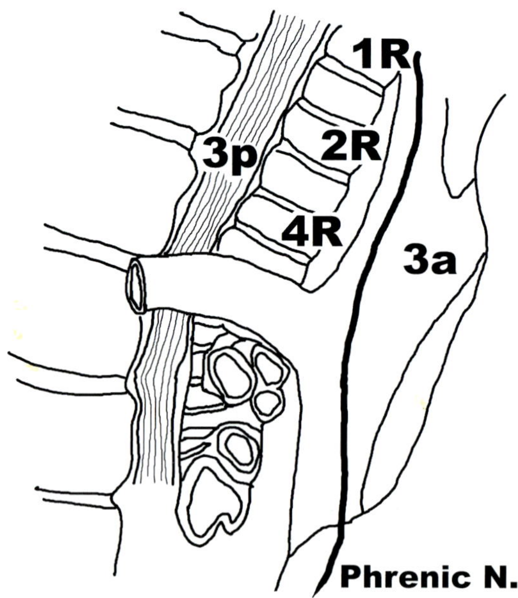

Fig. 2. Level 3 nodes: Mountain-Dresler thoracic lymph node map. Lateral view from right hemithorax. Note position of esophagus posterior to trachea and the relation of lymph node stations 3p and 1, 2, and 4R. (*Data from* Mountain CF. Revisions in the international system for staging lung cancer. Chest 1997;111(6):1710–7.)

Table 1
Naruke versus Mountain-Dresler lymph node stations

Japanese/Naruke	American Thoracic Society/Mountain-Dresler
Level 1	Levels 1 and 2
Levels 2, 3, 4R, 4L	Levels 4R, 4L
Levels 7 and 10	Level 7

Data from Rusch V, Crowley J, Giroux DJ, et al. The IASLC lung cancer staging project: proposals for the revision of the N descriptors in the forthcoming seventh edition of the TNM classification for lung cancer. J Thorac Oncol 2007;2:603–12.

example, cervical mediastinoscopy can be expected to biopsy the lymphatic material immediately inferior to the carina and along the left mainstem and right mainstem bronchus for 1 to 2 cm, level 7 in the Mountain-Dresler map and levels 7 and 10 in the Naruke map. Cervical mediastinoscopy is unlikely to reach the Mountain-Dresler level 10 lymph nodes, because they are too far out in the hilum. Adoption of a single system used worldwide would alleviate this confusion. In this article the Mountain-Dresler lymph node map is used.

Noninvasive staging

Noninvasive staging techniques, unlike invasive staging, do not provide tissue for pathologic evaluation. A recent American College of Chest Physicians consensus statement reported a pooled sensitivity of 51% and specificity of 85% for chest CT. More importantly, depending on the prevalence of lymph node disease in the population scanned, approximately 40% of nodes deemed malignant by chest CT will be benign, and 20% of all nodes deemed benign will be malignant. PET scanning has an average sensitivity of 74% and specificity of 84% [19], making PET scanning more sensitive than chest CT. In both cases, the possibility of false positives requires abnormal findings to be confirmed by tissue biopsy. No patient should be excluded from curative treatment on the basis of chest CT and PET alone. The only exception is the overwhelming presence of clinical and radiographic evidence of extrathoracic metastases. Although chest CT and PET rarely stand on their own in staging the N2 lymph nodes, they can assist greatly in choosing the method of biopsy, as discussed later in this article.

Cervical mediastinoscopy

The procedure

Cervical mediastinoscopy is performed under general anesthesia. A 1- to 2-cm incision is made in the neck just superior to the sternal notch. (Figs. 3, 4). The trachea is exposed, and a plane is established just anterior to the trachea (pretracheal fascia). This plane can be developed down to the level of the carina. Lymph node material is visualized and biopsied. Mediastinoscopy offers the ability to visualize lymphatic material directly and to distinguish nodes from the primary tumor mass. Sample sizes can range from small pieces of the lymph node, to the entire node, or to a complete dissection and removal of all nodes in that station, depending on patient characteristics and the surgeon's expertise (Fig. 5) [20,21].

Stations obtainable with cervical mediastinoscopy:

1L, 1R: highest mediastinal
2L, 2R: upper paratracheal
4L, 4R: lower paratracheal
7: subcarinal
10R, 10L: hilar (sometimes obtainable)

Stations not obtainable:

3: pre- and postvascular
5: aortopulmonary window
6: aortic arch
8: paraesophageal

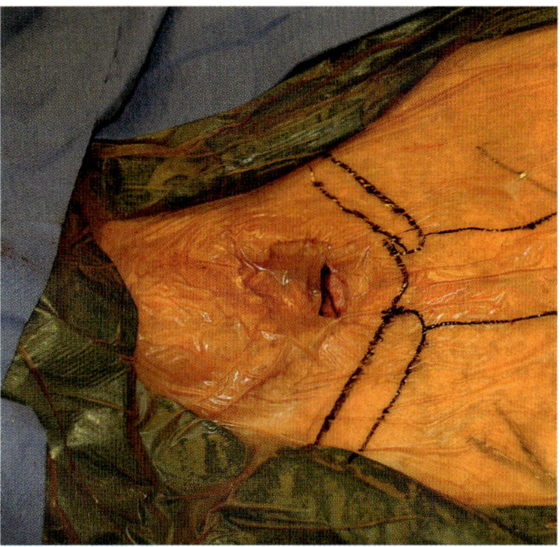

Fig. 3. Cervical mediastinoscopy incision. Head is to the left, feet are to the right; clavicle and sternum are drawn on the skin.

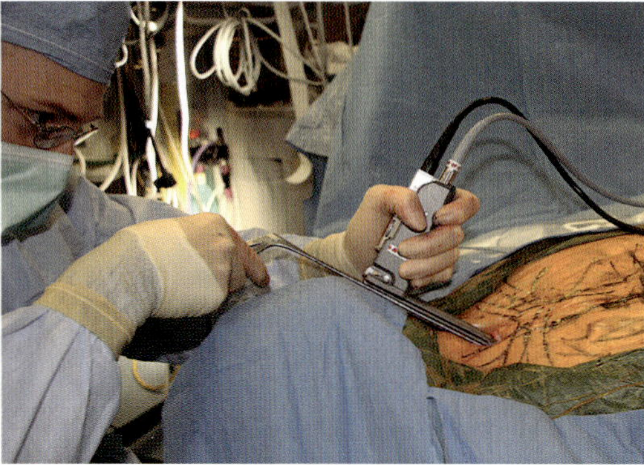

Fig. 4. Cervical mediastinoscopy and biopsy. Mediastinoscopy is being performed with a video and direct-vision mediastinoscope. Level 4R lymph nodes are being biopsied.

9: inferior pulmonary ligament
11 to 14: interlobar, lobar, segmental, subsegmental

What does it cost the patient?

Cervical mediastinoscopy has a morbidity of 2% and a mortality rate of 0.08% [22,23]. In a series of 2145 patients undergoing mediastinoscopy at Duke University between 1996 and 2005, 23 patients (0.05%) experienced complications. The most common complications were vocal cord dysfunction (0.55%), hemorrhage (0.33%), tracheal injury (0.09%), and pneumothorax (0.09%) [22]. One patient in the Duke study died (0.05%). Hammoud and colleagues [23] at Washington University in St. Louis reported a similar experience in 2137 cervical mediastinoscopies performed between 1988 and 1998. Complications occurred in 0.6% of patients, and death from the mediastinoscopy occurred in 0.05%. With more than 2 decades and more than 6000 cases of experience reported in the literature, cervical mediastinoscopy has a morbidity of about 1% and a mortality of 1 in 2000. It should be noted that the number of cases of EBUS, EUS, and thoracoscopy for lymph node staging reported in the literature are not large enough to detect such low morbidity and mortality rates, and therefore it is not known whether these modalities have a lower, higher, or similar rate of morbidity and mortality.

Most centers in the United States can perform cervical mediastinoscopy as ambulatory surgery, with the patient returning home the same day.

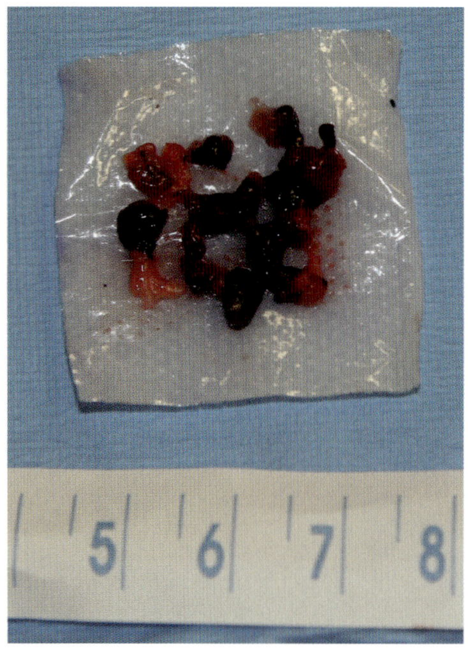

Fig. 5. Cervical mediastinoscopy biopsy specimen. Amount and biopsy size are typical of material biopsied from one lymph node station. Other stations would have similar biopsies. Measuring tape in centimeters.

Limitations

Cervical mediastinoscopy is best performed in a "virgin" plane. Radiation to the neck or mediastinum, previous neck surgery, and previous mediastinoscopy are all relative contraindications. For mediastinoscopy to be performed and visualization obtained, patients need to be able to extend the neck into a sniffing position. Cervical kyphosis, previous cervical spine surgery (especially fixation), or a severely obese neck can prevent adequate cervical extension. The introduction of the video mediastinoscope has lessened the amount of extension needed.

Bonus information

The external aspect of the anterior trachea and left and right mainstem bronchi can be evaluated for tumor involvement. For example, a medial right upper lobe neoplasm may appear radiographically immediately adjacent to the right side of the trachea. Invasion of the external aspect of the wall of the trachea can be determined with the mediastinoscope. Mediastinoscopy also can loosen the anterior tracheal plane to allow a tension-free anastomosis in preparation for a bronchoplastic procedure.

Test performance

The average false-negative rate of mediastinoscopy is 11% [24]. Half of these cases were lymph nodes not accessible by the mediastinoscope [23,25–30]. Studies evaluating cervical mediastinoscopy are detailed in Table 2. In studies evaluating mediastinoscopy in clinical stages I through III, the false-negative rate was 10%. In studies evaluating mediastinoscopy in clinical stages II and III only, the false-negative rate was 13%. In studies evaluating mediastinoscopy in clinical stage I, the false-negative rate was 8%. The literature indicates that the performance of mediastinoscopy is robust and consistent across clinical stages, perhaps because of the increased sampling and sample size of each reachable nodal station afforded by mediastinoscopy (Figs. 5, 6).

Thoracoscopy

The procedure

Thoracoscopy typically is done with general anesthesia. One to three 1-cm incisions are made through the chest wall. A thoracoscope is introduced, and the pleural space is inspected. Generally, anything that can be visualized or palpated from the pleural space can be biopsied. The procedure is done with either single-lung ventilation or double-lung ventilation and carbon dioxide insufflation. The procedure can be performed bilaterally, but doing so requires a second set of three incisions on the opposite side. Thoracoscopic lobectomy with lymph node dissection or sampling is performed routinely at multiple centers. Station by station, a thoracoscopic lymph

Table 2
Performance of cervical mediastinoscopy

Study/Year	No. Patients	Patient Type	Sensitivity (%)	FN (%)	Prevalence (%)
Studies grouping clinical stage I, II, and III together					
Lemaire and colleagues/2006 [23]	2145	cI–III	86	5	24
Hammoud and colleagues/1999 [29]	1369	cI–III	85	8	36
Coughlin and colleagues/1985 [25]	1259	cI–III	92	3	29
Luke and colleagues/1986 [66]	1000	cI–III	85	9	39
De Leyn and colleagues/1996 [67]	500	cI–III	76	13	39
Lardinois/2003 [30]	181	cI–III	87	8	34
Brion and colleagues/1985 [68]	153	cI–III	67	15	35
Jolly and colleagues/1991 [69]	136	cI–III	92	9	54
Ratto and colleagues/1990 [70]	123	cI–III	88	6	33
Ebner and colleagues/1999 [71]	116	cI–III	81	18	50
Gdeedo and colleagues/1997 [27]	100	cI–III	78	9	32
Deneffe and colleagues/1983 [72]	124	cI–III	68	12	31
Aaby and colleagues/1995 [73]	57	cI–III	84	11	44
Subtotal	5118	cI–III	82	10	38
Studies evaluating clinical stage II and/or III					
Page and colleagues/1987 [74]	345	cII–III	73	20	48
Dillemans and colleagues/1994 [75]	331	cII, III	72	16	41
Kimura/2003 [76]	125	cII–III	85	8	36
Rıordain and colleagues/1991 [77]	74	cII–III	81	16	50
Venissac/2003 [78]	154	cIII	97	6	71
Subtotal	1029	cII–III	82	13	49
Studies evaluating only clinical stage I					
Choi and colleagues/2003 [60]	291	cI	44	9	15
Gurses/2002 [61]	67	cN0	40	7	15
Subtotal	358	cI	42	8	15
Total	6505	—	78	11	39

In these studies, a positive mediastinoscopy was not followed by further lymph node dissection or other reference-standard confirmation of the positive test. Consequently specificity and false positive rates cannot be determined.

Data from Detterbeck FC, Jantz MA, Wallace M, et al. Invasive mediastinal staging of lung cancer: ACCP evidence-based clinical practice guidelines. 2nd edition. Chest 2007;132(3 Suppl):202S–20S.

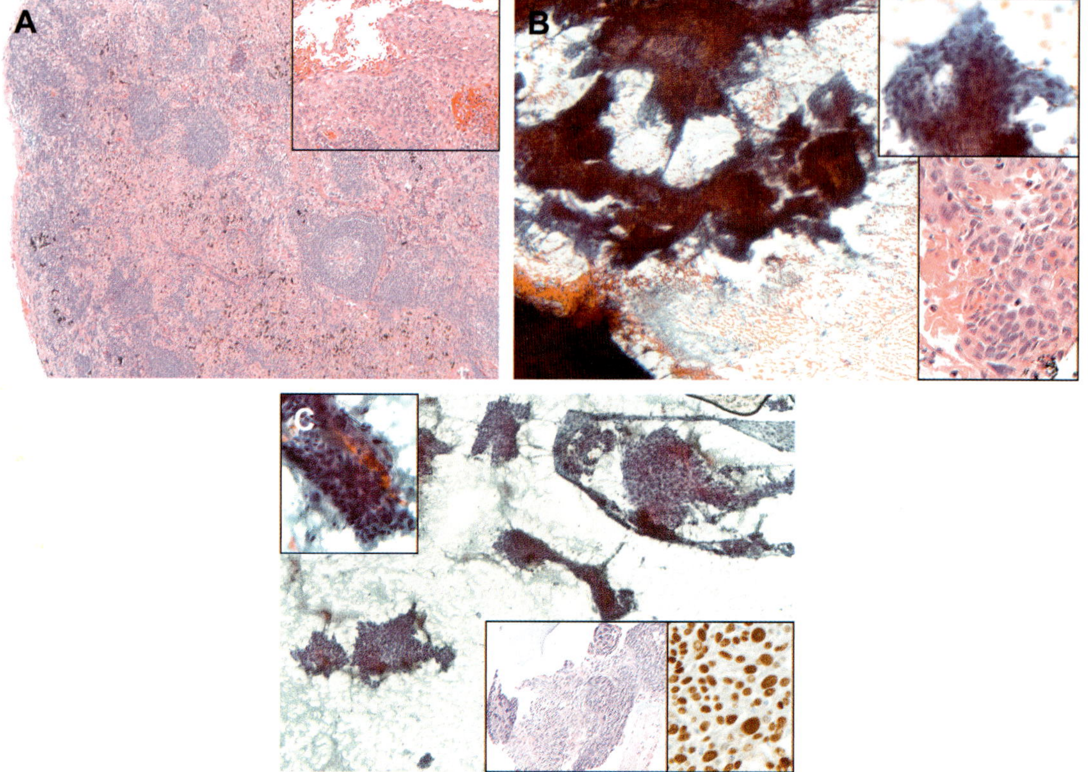

Fig. 6. Photomicrographs of typical histologic specimens from (*A*) cervical mediastinoscopy (original magnification, ×25 [inset ×400]) (*B*) EBUS-FNA (original magnification ×25 [inset top tight ×200; inset bottom right ×200]), and (*C*) EUS-FNA (original magnification ×25 [inset top right ×400; inset bottom middle ×200; inset bottom right ×630]). All three show biopsies of lymph nodes positive for squamous cell carcinoma. (*Courtesy of* D. Sauer, MD, Portland, OR.)

node dissection has been shown to be as complete as thoracotomy and lymphadenectomy [31–33].

Stations obtainable with left thoracoscopy:

- 5: aorto-pulmonary window
- 6: aortic arch
- 7: subcarinal
- 8L: left paraesophageal
- 9L: left inferior pulmonary ligament
- 10L: left hilar
- 11L to 14L: left lobar to parenchymal (sometimes obtainable)

Stations obtainable with right thoracoscopy:

- 3: anterior and posterior vascular
- 4R: right paratracheal
- 7: subcarinal
- 8R: right paraesophageal
- 9R: right inferior pulmonary ligament
- 10R: right hilar
- 11R to 14R: right lobar to parenchymal (sometimes obtainable)

Stations not obtainable:

- No lymph node station designated "right" or "left" (eg, 2R, 2L, 4R, 4L, 8R, 8L, 9R, 9L, 10–14R, 10–14L) can be obtained from a contralateral thorascopic approach.
- Station 3 cannot be obtained from a left-sided approach.
- Stations 5 and 6 cannot be obtained from a right-sided approach.
- 4L is very difficult to obtain from a left-sided approach and generally is considered not reachable thoracoscopically.
- Station 7 is obtainable from either side but is more difficult from the left.

Bonus information

Of the lymph node staging modalities discussed, thoracoscopy has the potential to yield the greatest additional information. Suspect lung nodules can be biopsied. The parietal and visceral pleura can be inspected, and any suspicious areas can have a directed biopsy. Unsuspected pleural studding is reported in approximately 4% of cases (range, 0–5%) [34]. In addition, 60% of cytologically negative pleural effusions have been shown by thoracoscopy to be caused by malignant pleural involvement [35].

Thoracoscopy also provides an opportunity for evaluating tumor stage, in particular the direct invasion of structures that precludes resection (T4). Up to 40% of patients who have radiographic evidence of T4 involvement have been down-staged (involvement not truly present) by thoracoscopy [35–37].

What does it cost the patient?

No mortality has been reported from thoracoscopic mediastinal staging. In eight studies reporting on 669 patients, 12 complications were reported (average 2%; range 0–9%) [34–41]. Many centers can perform a thoracoscopic mediastinal staging and discharge the patient home the same day or the next morning.

Limitations

In general, to tolerate thoracoscopy a patient must tolerate one-lung ventilation during the period of the procedure. Patients who have limited pulmonary reserve may not tolerate one lung ventilation long enough to complete the procedure. Previous thoracotomy, thoracoscopy, or pleurodesis can make the procedure more difficult but are not absolute contraindications. Thoracoscopic lysis of adhesions is possible.

Test performance

The false-negative rate for thoracoscopic lymph node evaluation is 15% in patients who have both enlarged and normal-sized nodes [24]. In studies evaluating only enlarged mediastinal lymph nodes, the false-negative rate remains 15%. In one study evaluating only normal-sized lymph nodes, the false-negative rate was 32%. This study was a prospective, multi-institutional study. In this population the prevalence of disease was 11%, suggesting that the false-negative rate depends to some degree on the prevalence of the disease in the studied population. Studies evaluating mediastinal lymph nodes thoracoscopically are itemized in Table 3.

Endobronchial ultrasound and needle aspiration biopsy

The procedure

EBUS and needle aspiration (EBUS-NA) generally is performed under general anesthesia with an endotracheal tube or laryngeal mask airway. A few centers perform EBUS with topical anesthesia and sedation [42,43]. The EBUS equipment consists of a bronchoscope 6 mm in diameter with a curvilinear ultrasound probe mounted to the front (Fig. 7). The scope has a working port and camera facing 30° off the long axis. Visualization through the EBUS scope is not as good as through a standard video bronchoscope because of the need to reduce the size of the video component to make room for the ultrasound probe in the tip of the scope. For this reason, fiberoptic bronchoscopy generally is performed first with a standard scope to clear secretions and evaluate the endobronchial airway. Any suspicious lesions are biopsied. The EBUS scope then is inserted, the balloon at its tip is inflated, and the ultrasound portion of the procedure is performed. All nodal stations viewable are evaluated systematically. Special attention is given to locating suspect nodes identified on the preoperative imaging. Vascular structures can be identified by their pulsatile appearance or, if there is doubt, by the application of color Doppler. Once all target lymph node tissue is identified, a specially designed needle housed in a sheath extending out the end of the scope to a preset distance is advanced through the scope . Ultrasound again is used to identify the target nodal tissue, and the needle is advanced through the wall of the airway and into the lymph node. Suction is placed on the needle, and the needle is passed through the lymph node multiple times (5–10) to obtain as good a sampling as possible (Fig. 8). The needle is pulled back into the sheath, and the sheath is removed. Aspirated material is fixed on a slide for immediate evaluation (Fig. 9).

Stations obtainable:

1L, 1R: highest mediastinal
2L, 2R: upper paratracheal
3: prevascular and retrotracheal
4L, 4R: lower paratracheal
7: subcarinal
10R, 10L: hilar
11L, 11R: interlobar

Table 3
Performance of thoracoscopic mediastinal lymph node biopsy/evaluation

Study/Year	No. of Patients	Patient Type	Sensitivity (%)	FN (%)	Prevalence (%)
Studies grouping all stages together					
Sebastian-Quetglas and colleagues/ 2003 [36]	105	All	37	20	29
Roberts and colleagues/1999 [40]	50	All	38	11	16
Subtotal	155		38	15	25
	–		–		
Studies evaluating clinical N2 disease					
Sebastian-Quetglas and colleagues/ 2003 [36]	30	cN2	50	58	73
Eggeling and colleagues/2002 [37]	73	cN2, cT4	99	4	70
Massone and colleagues/2003 [34]	53	cN2	100	0	64
Landreneau and colleagues/1993 [39]	33	cN2	100	0	42
Subtotal	—	189	87	15	64
Studies evaluating clinical N0 disease					
Sebastian-Quetglas and colleagues/ 2003 [36]	75	cN0	0	32	11
Total	–	419	75	7	44

A positive thoracoscopy was not followed by further lymph node dissection or other reference-standard confirmation of the positive test. Consequently specificity and false Positive rates cannot be determined.

Data from Detterbeck FC, Jantz MA, Wallace M, et al. Invasive mediastinal staging of lung cancer: ACCP evidence-based clinical practice guidelines. 2nd edition. Chest 2007;132(3 Suppl):202S–20S.

Stations not obtainable:

5: aortopulmonary window
6: aortic arch
8L, 8R: paraesophageal
9L, 9R: inferior pulmonary ligament
12–14: lobar and intralobar

What does it cost the patient?

In six studies reporting on 918 patients, no mortalities were reported. Most studies do not report complications related to EBUS. In studies reporting complications, complications included cough, shortening of the procedure because of patient discomfort, and a self-limited (30 cm^3) hemorrhage. All these complications occurred in catheter-based EBUS in which ultrasound was used to examine the airway and then was removed to allow placement of the biopsy needle, not in a real-time ultrasound and biopsy system [24].

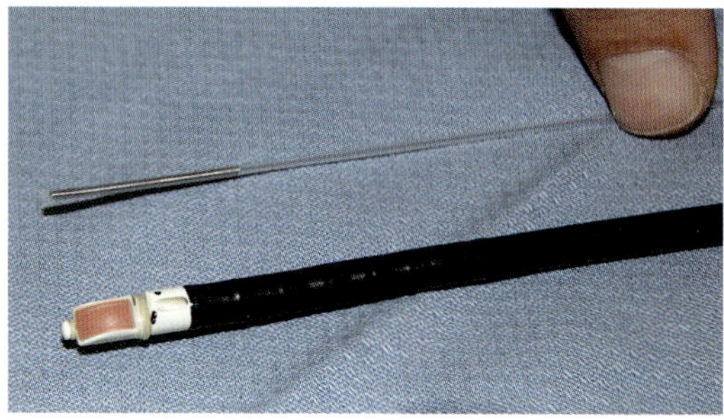

Fig. 7. EBUS aspiration needle (*top*) and he needle withdrawn into the sheath (*bottom*).

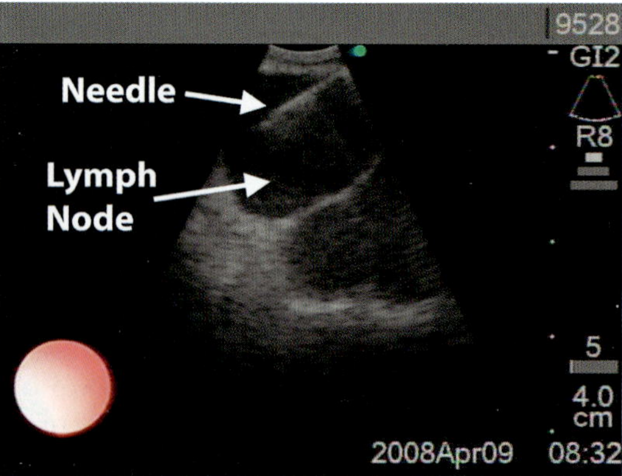

Fig. 8. EBUS of a 10R lymph node undergoing needle aspiration biopsy.

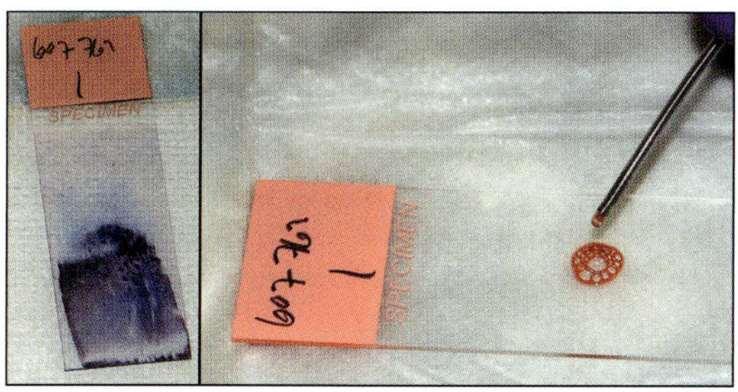

Fig. 9. Specimen and prepared smear from the 10R lymph node sampled in Fig. 8.

Limitations

Although multiple authors report performing EBUS using local anesthesia and sedation [42–46], general anesthesia is used at many institutions, including Oregon Health and Sciences University. The authors find that using general anesthesia, so there is no risk of cough or patient movement, increases their ability to perform a good examination and obtain biopsies. The ability to obtain biopsies of distal lymph nodes (station 11, interlobar) depends on the size of a patient's lobar airways and the ability to pass the EBUS scope into these airways.

Bonus information

EBUS can provide anatomic relations and tumor-staging information in a limited area around the central airways. Radial EBUS at 20 MHz has a spatial resolution of less than 1 mm and a depth of penetration of 4 to 5 cm. Real-time EBUS operates at a frequency of 7.5 MHz. This lower frequency improves depth of penetration at the cost of spatial resolution. Using a 20-MHz radial EBUS probe through the working channel of a standard bronchoscope, Herth and colleagues [47] examined 105 patients who had a tumor next to the trachea or within the tracheobronchial angles (central tumors) who then went on to surgical exploration. They evaluated the tumors for invasion into the airway versus compression without invasion. All lesions with visible tumor growth into the lumen were excluded. EBUS was able to predict the findings at surgery with no false positives and an 11% false-negative rate [47]. This performance was much better than the false-positive rate of almost 75% and false-negative rate of 25% seen with chest CT. Thus EBUS shows promise in yielding good tumor-staging information previously available at only the time of surgical exploration.

Test performance

The average false-negative rate of EBUS is 15%, as calculated from the systematic review of Detterbeck and colleagues [24] plus studies published since that review between July 2006 and April 2008. Detterbeck and colleagues [24] report an average false-negative rate of 24%. EBUS is still a relatively new technology, and the experience and literature are maturing. Most EBUS studies were performed in populations with relatively high disease prevalence—patients who had radiographically enlarged lymph nodes. Because it is less invasive, EBUS may be a good first-choice procedure in this population; however, because of the higher false-negative rate, any negative biopsy needs to be confirmed by cervical mediastinoscopy. Studies detailing the performance of EBUS-NA are detailed in Table 4. A combination of EBUS and EUS-NA allows a greater number of lymph node stations to be accessed. Wallace and colleagues [48] found false-negative rates of 12% for EBUS-NA alone and also for EUS-NA alone, but in the same setting the false-negative rate for both procedures was 3%. This study was done in a clinically very diverse group of patients (ie, patients ultimately found to not have cancer to stage III) in which the prevalence of N2 disease was 30%; the study points out that the NA techniques may be complementary.

Endoscopic esophageal ultrasound and needle-aspiration biopsy

The procedure

Most EUS-NA can be performed with conscious sedation. Unlike thoracoscopy and cervical mediastinoscopy, which rely on direct visualization of structures to identify lymph node stations, and EBUS, which relies heavily on the relation of the trachea and main airways to identify lymph node stations, EUS relies heavily on ultrasound identification of vascular structures and airways to locate stations. This reliance is necessary because there are few visual clues within the esophagus to identify appropriately what lies external to the esophagus. The distance from the incisors can be used as a gross approximation but should not be relied upon solely. The carina is located at about 27 to 30 cm from the incisors. Also important to note is the laterality of sampled lymph nodes. With

Table 4
Performance of endobronchial ultrasound with needle aspiration biopsy

Study/year	No. of Patients	Patient type	Sensitivity (%)	FN (%)	Prevalence (%)
Real-time ultrasound during needle biopsy technique					
Herth and colleagues/2006 [79]	502	C I-III	94	(89)	98
Yasufuku and colleagues/2005 [43]	108	cII–III	95	11	69
Yasufuku and colleagues/2004 [80]	70	cII–III	95	10	67
Vilmann and colleagues/2005 [81]	31	cII–III	85	28	65
Rintoul and colleagues/2005 [45]	20	cII–III	79	30	70
Yasufuku and colleagues/2006[a] [82]	102	cII-III	92	3	25
Wallace and colleagues/2008[a] [48]	97	c0-III	69	12	30
Vincent and colleagues/2008[a] [83]	113	cI-III	99	3	77
Subtotal	930	–	89	14	–
Catheter probe technique					
Kanoh and colleagues/2005 [44]	54	cII–III	86	37	81
Plat and colleagues/2006 [46]	33	cII–III	93	25	82
Subtotal	87	–	90	31	–
No mediastinal adenopathy (lymph node 0.5–1cm)					
Herth and colleagues/2006 [42]	100	cI	94	1	17
Herth and colleagues/2008[a] [63]	97	cI	89	1	9
Subtotal	197	–	92	1	–
Totals	1214	–	90	15	68

[a] Studies added to previously published systematic analysis. These studies span July 2006 to April 2008. Original averages from Detterbeck and colleagues were FN (% = 20), number of patients = 918, sensitivity = 90%. A positive EBUS-NA was not followed by further lymph node dissection or other reference standard confirmation of the positive tests.

Data from Detterbeck FC, Jantz MA, Wallace M, et al. Invasive mediastinal staging of lung cancer: ACCP evidence-based clinical practice guidelines. 2nd edition. Chest 2007;132(3 Suppl):202S–20S.

a right lower lobe cancer, a positive right level 8 or 9 lymph node is an N2 node, whereas a positive left level 8 or 9 lymph node is an N3 node. A typical EUS will advance the echoendoscope to about 35 cm from the incisors.

The descending aorta is identified. With the aorta kept in view, advancing the scope to approximately 45 cm should visualize the celiac axis bifurcation. Rotating the scope clockwise (to the patient's left) will show the left adrenal. The scope then is withdrawn, visualizing first the inferior pulmonary ligament lymph nodes (9L and 9R) and then the periesophageal lymph nodes (8L and 8R), the subcarinal lymph nodes (7), and the level 3p lymph nodes. Located more anteriorly, next to the trachea on the right and left at the same level as the 3p lymph nodes, are the lower paratracheal lymph nodes (4R and 4L) and upper paratracheal lymph nodes (2R and 2L). The subcarinal space is located about 27 to 30 cm from the incisors and is bounded inferiorly by the left atrium and superiorly by the right main pulmonary artery [49]. The 4L lymph nodes are located between the arch of the aorta, the main pulmonary artery, and the midline of the trachea. The aortopulmonary window lymph nodes are located lateral to the ligamentum arteriosum (see Fig. 1). Whether the anteroposterior window lymph nodes can be sampled via EUS is controversial, because the esophagus is located several centimeters away from these nodes with the aorta and pulmonary artery interposed. Also controversial is whether the 2R and 4R lymph nodes can be reached, because the lymph node station immediately adjacent to the esophagus is level 3p (see Fig. 2), and 2R and 4R nodes are located more anterior, lateral and anterior to the trachea. Once a suspect node is identified, fine-needle aspiration (FNA) is performed much like EBUS. Unlike EBUS, EUS has the option of biopsy with a 22-gauge FNA or a 19-gauge core biopsy. The first yields a smear that is read for cytology; the second yields tissue that can yield histology (see Fig. 6C).

Stations obtainable:

2L, 2R: upper paratracheal (difficult to reach with EUS)
3p: retrotracheal

4L, 4R: lower paratracheal (difficult to reach with EUS)
7: subcarinal
8L, 8R: paraesophageal
9L, 9R: inferior pulmonary ligament

Stations not obtainable:

3a: prevascular
5: aortopulmonary window
6: aortic
10–14: hilar, lobar, and parenchymal

What does it cost the patient?

EUS seems to have a low complication rate. Many studies using EUS in lung cancer do not report complication rates, however. Only one complication, a transient fever, was reported in 369 patients in six studies reporting complications. EUS is performed on an outpatient basis requiring sedation and a day off work but no overnight hospitalization [50–54].

Evaluation of 3324 patients undergoing EUS and EUS-FNA for all comers (51% benign and 49% malignant including lung cancer in 8.9%) found mortality of 0.06% and a morbidity rate of 0.3%. All morbidities were in patients who had esophageal cancer or pancreatic pathologies, and all mortalities were in patients who had pancreatic pathologies [55].

Limitations

Most currently available echoendoscopes have a tip diameter ranging from 1.2 cm to 1.5 cm [56] and cannot be used in patients whose esophagus is narrowed by strictures to a diameter smaller than this. Real-time EBUS scopes have an outer diameter of 6 mm and have been used in the esophagus.

Bonus information

Endoscopic esophagoscopy allows evaluation of the left adrenal gland and left lobe of the liver. EUS can biopsy suspect lesions in the left adrenal gland. Because ultrasound cannot penetrate air-filled structures, visualization of many primary tumors and their surroundings is not possible. By definition, however, a primary lesion seen on EUS has no intervening air-filled lung and is abutting the parietal pleural. Irregularities in this interface have been used as an indicator of invasion. Based on this type of evaluation, Varadarajulu and colleagues [57] evaluated 175 patients for tumor stage by EUS who later went on to confirmatory evaluation by thoracoscopy or thoracotomy. They found a 30% false-positive rate and a 1% false-negative rate. The false positives were lesions read as T4 on EUS found on surgical exploration to be T3 and T2 lesions. Clearly, great caution should be taken in denying patients curative therapies based on EUS T staging alone [57]. EUS can identify pleural effusions that then can be sampled via EUS-FNA for cytology.

Test performance

EUS-FNA has an average false-negative rate of 16%, as calculated from the systematic review of Detterbeck and colleagues [24] plus studies published since that review between July 2006 and April 2008. Detterbeck and colleagues [24] report an average false-negative rate of 19%. EUS-FNA is one of the few modalities in which positive biopsies have been studied further, allowing determination of a false-positive rate. In one study, 80 patients underwent EUS-FNA, mediastinoscopy, and thoracotomy. In two patients, metastatic disease that was identified in the subcarinal lymph nodes was not found after a complete subcarinal lymphadenectomy, for a false-positive rate of 7%. The authors believe the primary tumor was sampled inadvertently and labeled as a subcarinal lymph node [58]. A second study by Wiersema and colleagues [53] found a false-positive rate of 4%. In studies evaluating only enlarged lymph nodes, the false-negative rate averaged 22%. In studies evaluating normal-sized lymph nodes, the false-negative rate averaged 14%. These studies, however, showed a disease prevalence of 36% for this population, whereas a prevalence of 20% to 25% would be expected. Some other selection criteria were used, possibly PET avidity, to screen candidates for EUS-FNA better within the subcentimeter lymph node group. It has been shown that EUS-FNA can locate and sample lymph nodes smaller than 1 cm [51,54]. Studies detailing the performance of EUS-FNA are given in Table 5.

Choosing which procedure to perform

The previous discussion indicates that each procedure has advantages and disadvantages. It also is clear that not all lymph nodes can be sampled by each procedure. A thoracic lymph

Table 5
Performance of endoscopic esophageal ultrasound with needle biopsy

Study/Year	No. of Patients	Patient Type	Sensitivity (%)	FN (%)	Prevalence (%)
EUS-NA studies that pooled all stages					
Annema and colleagues/2005 [58]	193	cN0–3	90	27	79
Annema and colleagues/2004 [84]	36	?	93	20	78
Caddy and colleagues/2005 [85]	33	?	91	15	67
Fritscher-Ravens and colleagues/2003 [51]	33	cN0–3	88	11	48
Larsen and colleagues/2005 [86]	55	cN0–3	92	6	47
Sawhney and colleagues/2007[a] [87]	44	cN0-3	50	7	14
Subtotal	394	cN0–3	84	14	55
EUS-NA studies in patients with radiographic adenopathy mediastinal nodes					
Wallace and colleagues/2001 [54]	107	cN2,3	87	32	79
Annema and colleagues/2005 [58]	93	cN2,3	71	15	38
Kramer and colleagues/2004 [88]	81	cN2,3	72	61	85
Wiersema and colleagues/2001 [53]	33	cN2,3	100	0	76
Larsen and colleagues/2002 [89]	29	cN2,3	90	18	69
Silvestri and colleagues/1996 [52]	26	cN2,3	88	18	65
Gress and colleagues/1997 [50]	24	cN2,3	93	10	63
Tournoy and colleagues/2008[a] [90]	75	cN2,3	96	33	92
Subtotal	493	cN2,3	87	23	71
EUS-NA studies in patients without mediastinal adenopathy					
Eloubeidi and colleagues/2005 [91–93]	104	cN0,1	93	4	38
Wallace and colleagues/2004 [57]	64	cN0,1	61	18	36
LeBlanc and colleagues/2005 [62]	67	cN0,1	45	21	33
Tournoy and colleagues/2008[a] [90]	25	cN0	93	8	56
Subtotal	270	cN0,1	73	13	41
Total	1157		81	16	59

[a] Studies spanning July 2006 to April 2008 added to the systematic analysis published by Detterbeck and colleagues [24]. Sensitivity = 84%, FN = 19%, prevalence = 61%.

Data from Detterbeck FC, Jantz MA, Wallace M, et al. Invasive mediastinal staging of lung cancer: ACCP evidence-based clinical practice guidelines. 2nd edition. Chest 2007;132(3 Suppl):202S–20S.

node map combining all four procedures and the nodes they can reach is shown in Fig. 10. An important consideration in choosing a modality is the pretest probability of disease in that patient. The goal of invasive staging for mediastinal disease is to confirm the absence of disease and to affirm that the next step in treatment, generally surgical resection, is appropriate. For this reason, the false-negative rate is the most useful measure. A second consideration is the lack of data on false-positive rates. A biopsy positive for neoplasm is a relatively strong finding, because the tumor cells are present under the microscope. In this situation aA false-positive result generally does not occur, because the pathologist has misinterpreted a benign specimen as malignant. Rather, false positives seem to occur and to affect patient care through the incorrect identification of where a biopsy was taken. Incorrectly identifying an N1 node as an N2 node (hilar versus mediastinal), the biopsy of a primary tumor as a nodal biopsy, or an ipsilateral node as a contralateral node (N2

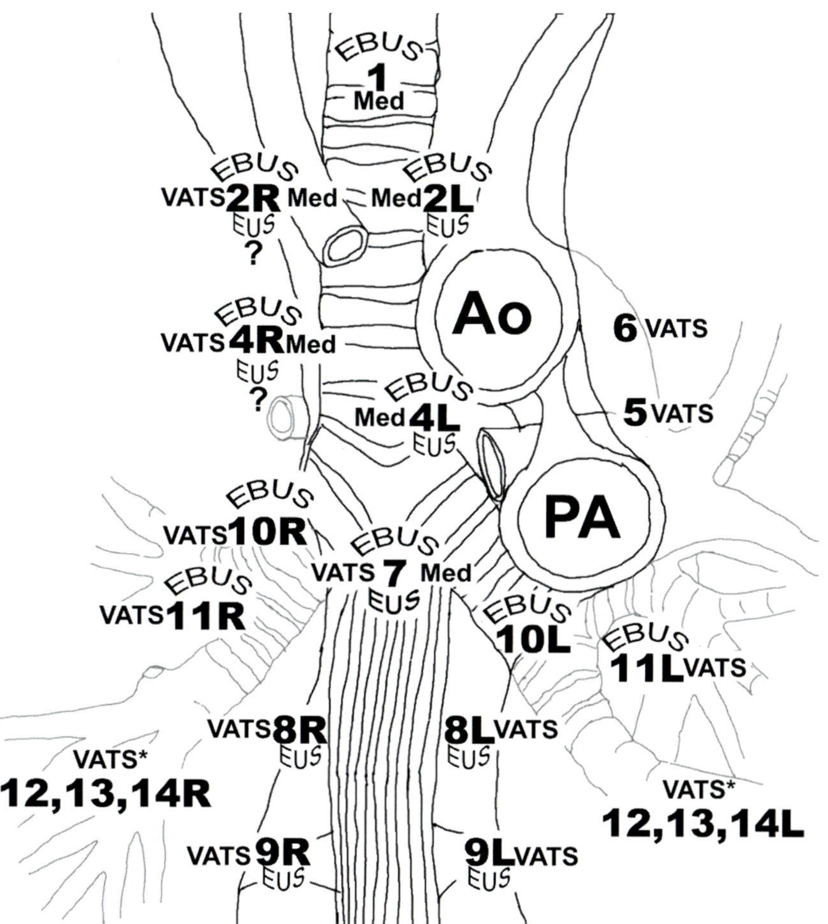

Fig. 10. Biopsy procedures used at various lymph nodes levels. Ao, aorta; EBUS, endobronchial ultrasound and needle aspiration; EUS, endoscopic ultrasound and needle aspiration; Med, cervical mediastinoscopy and biopsy; PA, pulmonary artery; VATS, thoracoscopy and biopsy; ?, 2R and 4R lymph node stations are quite anterior and can be difficult to reach with EUS. *, VATS can obtain intraparenchymal lymph nodes but only with either extensive dissection of the lung or a wedge resection including lymphatic material and pulmonary parenchyma.

versus N3) are all possible sources of error. In these instances, the patient would be overstaged and might not receive curative therapies. In studies that followed up a positive biopsy with further reference-standard assessment, the false-positive rates hovered around 6%. It is the clinician's responsibility to understand clearly where nodal tissue was obtained, especially in relation to the primary tumor, and to insist that nodal stations not obtained personally be labeled appropriately.

A method of predicting the prevalence of disease in a population based on radiographic imaging is presented by Detterbeck and colleagues [24,59]. Using chest CT, four groups can be categorized. In the first group are patients who have extensive mediastinal infiltration. These patients do not require invasive staging, because the radiographic evidence usually is considered adequate. These patients do require biopsy to confirm the tumor type, but this biopsy can be obtained from whichever location is easiest.

In the second group are patients who have discrete enlarged mediastinal lymph nodes. Because the false-positive rates are 40% for chest CT and 15% to 20% for PET, patients who have radiographically positive lymph nodes should undergo confirmation of disease by invasive testing. The procedure chosen will depend on several variables. First, as mentioned earlier, the node that is enlarged must be approachable by the selected technique. Second, not all techniques will be available at all centers. It also is likely that not all centers will be able to achieve the performance characteristics reported in the literature and that, because of personnel or interest levels, centers will develop expertise in select procedures, making these procedures safer and more effective. As reported in the literature, all techniques are relatively equal in terms of morbidity and mortality. Thoracoscopy and cervical mediastinoscopy require an incision and can be considered slightly more invasive than the NA techniques. An NA biopsy is a good first start, but in general, because of the high-false negative rate (averaging 25% to 30%) of NA techniques, any negative biopsy should be confirmed by cervical mediastinoscopy.

In the third group are patients who have non-enlarged mediastinal lymph nodes but who have central tumors or evidence of positive N1 lymph nodes. These patients have been found to harbor radiographically occult disease in the N2 lymph nodes approximately 20% of the time. In this patient population cervical mediastinoscopy has a well-established track record with low false-negative rates ranging from 7% to 9% [60,61]. The false-negative rate of EUS-FNA is higher, ranging 14% to 21% [24,54,59,62]. Although in early studies EBUS generally was used to evaluate enlarged lymph nodes, it has been used to evaluate subcentimeter lymph nodes (0.5–1 cm) with promising results [42,63]. Cervical mediastinoscopy remains the reference standard in this population, but the NA techniques (EBUS and EUS) can be considered as initial studies. Negative studies still should be confirmed by cervical mediastinoscopy.

In the final group are patients who have peripheral tumors and no radiographic adenopathy. The false-negative rate of chest CT in this group is 10% [59]. The addition of a negative PET scan lowers the false-negative rate to 5% [64]. It can be argued that invasive staging is not needed in this group. Lymph node sampling or dissection should be performed at the time of definitive surgical procedure.

Summary

In 2005 the American College of Surgeons conducted a survey examining lung cancer practice patterns at 729 hospitals in the United States. In 11,668 surgically treated patients, 92% received a preoperative chest CT. Only 27% of these patients underwent mediastinoscopy, and lymph node material was sampled in less than half of these patients. At the time of surgical resection, additional mediastinal lymph nodes were sampled in only 58% of patients. In the remaining 42% only the lymph node material attached to the surgical specimen (N1 nodes) was sampled [65]. Although this article discusses the finer points of the minimally invasive evaluation of the N2 lymph nodes, any procedure to evaluate these nodes is better than simply ignoring them.

Acknowledgments

The authors thank Jill Rose for her assistance in preparing and editing this article.

References

[1] Robinson LA, Ruckdeschel JC, Wagner H Jr, et al. Treatment of non-small cell lung cancer-stage IIIA: ACCP evidence-based clinical practice guidelines. 2nd edition. Chest 2007;132(3 Suppl):243S–65S.

[2] Rosell R, Gomez-Codina J, Camps C, et al. Preresectional chemotherapy in stage IIIA non-small-cell lung cancer: a 7-year assessment of a randomized controlled trial. Lung Cancer 1999;26:7–14.

[3] Rosell R, Gomez-Codina J, Camps C, et al. A randomized trial comparing preoperative chemotherapy plus surgery with surgery alone in patients with non-small-cell lung cancer. N Engl J Med 1994;330:153–8.

[4] Roth JA, Fossella F, Komaki R, et al. A randomized trial comparing perioperative chemotherapy and surgery with surgery alone in resectable stage IIIA non-small-cell lung cancer. J Natl Cancer Inst 1994;86(9):673–80.

[5] Roth JA, Atkinson EN, Fossella F, et al. Long-term follow-up of patients enrolled in a randomized trial comparing perioperative chemotherapy and surgery with surgery alone in resectable stage IIIA non-small-cell lung cancer. Lung Cancer 1998;21(1):1–6.

[6] Pass H, Pogrebniak H, Steinberg S, et al. Randomized trial of neoadjuvant therapy for lung cancer: interim analysis. Ann Thorac Surg 1992;53:992–8.

[7] Wagner H Jr, Lad T, Piantadosi S, et al. Randomized phase 2 evaluation of preoperative radiation therapy and preoperative chemotherapy with mitomycin, vinblastine, and cisplatin in patients with technically unresectable stage IIIA and IIIB non-small cell cancer of the lung: LCSG 881. Chest 1994;106(6 Suppl):348S–54S.

[8] Elias A, Herndon J, Kumar P, et al. A phase III comparison of "best local-regional therapy" with or without chemotherapy (CT) for stage IIIA T1-3N2 non-small cell lung cancer (NSCLC): preliminary results [abstract]. Proc Am Soc Clin Oncol Annu Meet 1997;16:448a.

[9] Depierre A, Milleron B, Moro-Sibilot D, et al. Preoperative chemotherapy followed by surgery compared with primary surgery in resectable stage I

(except T1N0), II, and IIIa non-small-cell lung cancer. J Clin Oncol 2002;20(1):247–53.

[10] Nagai K, Tsuchiya R, Mori T, et al. A randomized trial comparing induction chemotherapy followed by surgery with surgery alone for patients with stage IIIA N2 non-small cell lung cancer (JCOG 9209). J Thorac Cardiovasc Surg 2003;125(2):254–60.

[11] Garland L, Robinson L, Wagner H. Evaluation and management of patients with stage IIIA (N2) non-small-cell lung cancer. Chest Surg Clin N Am 2001;11:69–100, viii.

[12] Taylor NA, Liao ZX, Cox JD, et al. Equivalent outcome of patients with clinical stage IIIA non-small-cell lung cancer treated with concurrent chemoradiation compared with induction chemotherapy followed by surgical resection. Int J Radiat Oncol Biol Phys 2004;58(1):204–12.

[13] van Meerbeeck JP, Gaafar R, Manegold C, et al. Randomized phase III study of cisplatin with or without raltitrexed in patients with malignant pleural mesothelioma: an intergroup study of the European Organisation for Research and Treatment of Cancer Lung Cancer group and the National Cancer Institute of Canada. J Clin Oncol 2005;23(28):6881–9.

[14] Albain KS, Swann RS, Rusch VR, et al. Phase III study of concurrent chemotherapy and radiotherapy (CT/RT) vs CT/RT followed by surgical resection for stage IIIA(pN2) non-small cell lung cancer (NSCLC): outcomes update of North American Intergroup 0139 (RTOG 9309). J Clin Oncol (Meeting Abstracts) 2005;23(16 Suppl):7014.

[15] Mountain CF. A new international staging system for lung cancer. Chest 1986;89(4):225S–33S.

[16] Mountain CF. Revisions in the international system for staging lung cancer. Chest 1997;111(6):1710–7.

[17] Rusch V, Crowley J, Giroux DJ, et al. The IASLC lung cancer staging project: proposals for the revision of the N descriptors in the forthcoming seventh edition of the TNM classification for lung cancer. J Thorac Oncol 2007;2:603–12.

[18] Naruke T, Suemasu K, Ishikawa S. Lymph node mapping and curability at various levels of metastasis in resected lung cancer. J Thorac Cardiovasc Surg 1978;76:832–9.

[19] Silvestri GA, Gould MK, Margolis ML, et al. Noninvasive staging of non-small cell lung cancer: ACCP evidenced-based clinical practice guidelines. 2nd edition. Chest 2007;132(3 Suppl):178S–201S.

[20] Leschber G, Sperling D, Klemm W, et al. Does video-mediastinoscopy improve the results of conventional mediastinoscopy? Eur J Cardiothorac Surg 2008;33(2):289–93.

[21] Witte B, Hurtgen M. Video-assisted mediastinoscopic lymphadenectomy (VAMLA). Journal of Thoracic Oncology 2007;2:367–9.

[22] Kiser A, Detterbeck F. General aspects of surgical treatment. In: Detterbeck F, editor. Diagnosis and treatment of lung cancer: an evidence-based guide for the practicing clinician. Philadelphia: W.B. Saunders; 2001. p. 133–47.

[23] Lemaire A, Nikolic I, Petersen T, et al. Nine-year single center experience with cervical mediastinoscopy: complications and false negative rate. The Ann Thorac Surg 2006;82(4):1185–90.

[24] Detterbeck FC, Jantz MA, Wallace M, et al. Invasive mediastinal staging of lung cancer: ACCP evidence-based clinical practice guidelines. 2nd edition. Chest 2007;132(3 Suppl):202S–20S.

[25] Coughlin M, Deslauriers J, Beaulieu M, et al. Role of mediastinoscopy in pretreatment staging of patients with primary lung cancer. Ann Thorac Surg 1985;40:556–60.

[26] Staples CA, Muller NL, Miller RR, et al. Mediastinal nodes in bronchogenic carcinoma: comparison between CT and mediastinoscopy. Radiology 1988;167(2):367–72.

[27] Gdeedo A, et al. General aspects of surgical treatment. Prospective evaluation of computed tomography and mediastinoscopy in mediastinal lymph node staging. Eur Respir J 1997;10(7):1547–51.

[28] Van Den Bosch J, Gelissen H, Wagenaar S. Exploratory thoracotomy in bronchial carcinoma. J Thorac Cardiovasc Surg 1983;85:733–7.

[29] Hammoud Z, Anderson RC, Meyers BF, et al. The current role of mediastinoscopy in the evaluation of thoracic disease. J Thorac Cardiovasc Surg 1999;118:894–9.

[30] Lardinois D, Schallberger A, Betticher D, et al. Postinduction video-mediastinoscopy is as accurate and safe as video-mediastinoscopy in patients without pretreatment for potentially operable non-small cell lung cancer. Ann Thorac Surg 2003;75:1102–6.

[31] Watanabe A, Koyanagi T, Ohsawa H, et al. Systematic node dissection by VATS is not inferior to that through an open thoracotomy: a comparative clinicopathologic retrospective study. Surgery 2005;138:510–7.

[32] Ettinger DS, Bepler G, Bueno R, et al. Non-small cell lung cancer clinical practice guidelines in oncology. J Natl Compr Canc Netw 2006;4:548–82.

[33] Henschke CI, Wisnivesky J, Yankelevitz DF, et al. Small stage I cancers of the lung: genuineness and curability. Lung Cancer 2003;39:327–30.

[34] Massone P, Lequaglie C, Magnani B, et al. The real impact and usefulness of video-assisted thoracoscopic surgery in the diagnosis and therapy of clinical lymphadenopathies of the mediastinum. Ann Surg Oncol 2003;10:1197–202.

[35] De Giacomo T, Rendina EA, Venuta F, et al. Thoracoscopic staging of IIIb non-small cell lung cancer before neoadjuvant therapy. The Ann Thorac Surg 1997;64(5):1409–11.

[36] Sebastián-Quetglás F, Molins L, Baldó X, et al. Clinical value of video-assisted thoracoscopy for preoperative staging of non-small cell lung cancer: a prospective study of 105 patients. Lung Cancer 2003;42(3):297–301.

[37] Eggeling S, Martin T, Böttger J, et al. Invasive staging of non-small cell lung cancer—a prospective study. European Journal of Cardio-Thoracic Surgery 2002;22(5):679–84.

[38] Loscertales J, Jimenez-Merchan R, Arenas-Linares C, et al. The use of videoassisted thoracic surgery in lung cancer: evaluation of resectability in 296 patients and 71 pulmonary exeresis with radical lymphadenectomy. European Journal of Cardio-Thoracic Surgery 1997;12(6):892–7.

[39] Landreneau R, Hazelrigg SR, Mack MJ, et al. Thoracoscopic mediastinal lymph node sampling: useful for mediastinal lymph node stations inaccessible by cervical mediastinoscopy. J Thorac Cardiovasc Surg 1993;106:554–8.

[40] Roberts JR, Blum MG, Arildsen R, et al. Prospective comparison of radiologic, thoracoscopic, and pathologic staging in patients with early non-small cell lung cancer. The Ann Thorac Surg 1999;68(4): 1154–8.

[41] Wain J. Video-assisted thoracoscopy and the staging of lung cancer. Ann Thorac Surg 1993;56:776–8.

[42] Herth FJ, Ernst A, Eberhardt R, et al. Endobronchial ultrasound-guided transbronchial needle aspiration of lymph nodes in the radiologically normal mediastinum. Eur Respir J 2006;28(5):910–4.

[43] Yasufuku K, Chiyo M, Koh E, et al. Endobronchial ultrasound guided transbronchial needle aspiration for staging of lung cancer. Lung Cancer 2005; 50(3):347–54.

[44] Kanoh K, Miyazawa T, Kurimoto N, et al. Endobronchial ultrasonography guidance for transbronchial needle aspiration using a double-channel bronchoscope. Chest 2005;128(1):388–93.

[45] Rintoul RC, Skwarski KM, Murchison JT, et al. Endobronchial and endoscopic ultrasound-guided real-time fine-needle aspiration for mediastinal staging. Eur Respir J 2005;25(3):416–21.

[46] Plat G, Pierard P, Haller A, et al. Endobronchial ultrasound and positron emission tomography positive mediastinal lymph nodes. Eur Respir J 2006; 27(2):276–81.

[47] Herth F, Ernst A, Schulz M, et al. Endobronchial ultrasound reliably differentiates between airway infiltration and compression by tumor. Chest 2003; 123(2):458–62.

[48] Wallace MB, Pascual J, Raimondo M, et al. Minimally invasive endoscopic staging of suspected lung cancer. JAMA 2008;299:540–6.

[49] Eloubeidi MA. Endoscopic ultrasound-guided fine-needle aspiration in the staging and diagnosis of patients with lung cancer. Seminars in Thoracic and Cardiovascular Surgery 2007;19(206–11):206.

[50] Gress FG, Savides TJ, Sandler A, et al. Endoscopic ultrasonography, fine-needle aspiration biopsy guided by endoscopic ultrasonography, and computed tomography in the preoperative staging of non-small-cell lung cancer: a comparison study. Ann Intern Med 1997;127(8 Part 1):604–12.

[51] Fritscher-Ravens A, Soehendra N, Schirrow L, et al. Role of transesophageal endosonography-guided fine-needle aspiration in the diagnosis of lung cancer. Chest 2000;117(2):339–45.

[52] Silvestri GA, Hoffman BJ, Bhutani MS, et al. Endoscopic ultrasound with fine-needle aspiration in the diagnosis and staging of lung cancer. The Ann Thorac Surg 1996;61(5):1441–6.

[53] Wiersema MJ, Vazquez-Sequeiros E, Wiersema LM. Evaluation of mediastinal lymphadenopathy with endoscopic US-guided fine-needle aspiration biopsy. Radiology 2001;219(1):252–7.

[54] Wallace M, Silvestri GA, Sahai AV, et al. Endoscopic ultrasound-guided fine needle aspiration for staging patients with carcinoma of the lung. Ann Thorac Surg 2001;72:1861–7.

[55] Mortensen M, Fristrup C, Holm FS, et al. Prospective evaluation of patient tolerability, satisfaction with patient information, and complications in endoscopic ultrasonography. Endoscopy 2005;37: 146–53.

[56] Tierney WM, Adler DG, Chand B, et al. ASGE Technology Committee. Echoendoscopes. Gastrointest Endosc 2007;66(3):435–42.

[57] Varadarajulu S, Schmulewitz N, Wildi SM, et al. Accuracy of EUS in staging of T4 lung cancer. Gastrointest Endosc 2004;59(3):345–8.

[58] Annema JT, Versteegh MI, Veselic M, et al. Endoscopic ultrasound added to mediastinoscopy for preoperative staging of patients with lung cancer. JAMA 2005;294(8):931–6.

[59] Detterbeck F. Integration of mediastinal staging techniques for lung cancer. Seminars in Thoracic and Cardiovascular Surgery 2007;19(217–24):217.

[60] Choi Y, Shim YM, Kim J, et al. Mediastinoscopy in patients with clinical stage I non-small cell lung cancer. Ann Thorac Surg 2003;75:364–6.

[61] Gurses A, Turna A, Bedirhan MA, et al. The value of mediastinoscopy in preoperative evaluation of mediastinal involvement in non-small-cell lung cancer patients with clinical NO disease. Thorac Cardiovasc Surg 2002;50:174–7.

[62] LeBlanc JK, Devereaux BM, Imperiale TF, et al. Endoscopic ultrasound in non-small cell lung cancer and negative mediastinum on computed tomography. Am J Respir Crit Care Med 2005;171(2): 177–82.

[63] Herth FJ, Eberhardt R, Krasnik M, et al. Endobronchial ultrasound-guided transbronchial needle aspiration of lymph nodes in the radiologically and positron emission tomography-normal mediastinum in patients with lung cancer. Chest 2008;133(4): 887–91.

[64] Meyers BF, Haddad R, Siegel BA, et al. Cost-effectiveness of routine mediastinoscopy in computed tomography- and positron emission tomography-screened patients with stage I lung cancer. Journal of Thoracic and Cardiovascular Surgery 2006;131: 822–9.

[65] Little AG, Rusch VW, Bonner JA, et al. Patterns of surgical care of lung cancer patients. Ann Thorac Surg 2005;80:2051–6.

[66] Luke W, Pearson FG, Todd R, et al. Prospective evaluation of mediastinoscopy for assessment of carcinoma of the lung. J Thorac Cardiovasc Surg 1986; 91:53–6.

[67] De Leyn P, Schoonooghe P, Deneffe G, et al. Surgery for non-small cell lung cancer with unsuspected metastasis to ipsilateral mediastinal or subcarinal nodes (N2 disease). European Journal of Cardio-Thoracic Surgery 1996;10(8):649–55.

[68] Brion J, Hutchinson CH, Detterbeck F, et al. Role of computed tomography and mediastinoscopy in preoperative staging of lung carcinoma. J Comput Assist Tomogr 1985;9:480–4.

[69] Jolly P, Frola C, Cantoni S, et al. Routine computed tomographic scans, selective mediastinoscopy, and other factors in evaluation of lung cancer. J Thorac Cardiovasc Surg 1991;102:266–70.

[70] Ratto G, Marra A, Butturini E, et al. Improving clinical efficacy of computed tomographic scan in the preoperative assessment of patients with non-small cell lung cancer. J Thorac Cardiovasc Surg 1990;99:416–25.

[71] Ebner H, Lacquet LM, Gyselen A. Clinical value of cervical mediastinoscopy in the staging of bronchial carcinoma. Ann Ital Chir 1999;70:873–9.

[72] Deneffe G, Lacquet L, Gyselen A. Cervical mediastinoscopy and anterior mediastinotomy in patients with lung cancer and radiologically normal mediastinum. Eur J Respir Dis 1983;64:613–9.

[73] Aaby C, Kristensen S, Nielsen S. Mediastinal staging of non-small-cell lung cancer: computed tomography and cervical mediastinoscopy. ORL J Otorhinolaryngol Relat Spec 1995;57:279–85.

[74] Page A, Deneffe G, Verschakelen J, et al. Surgical treatment of bronchogenic carcinoma: the importance of staging in evaluating late survival. Can J Surg 1987;30:96–9.

[75] Dillemans B, Deneffe G, Verschakelen J, et al. Value of computed tomography and mediastinoscopy in preoperative evaluation of mediastinal nodes in non-small cell lung cancer. A study of 569 patients. Eur J Cardiothorac Surg 1994;8:37–42.

[76] Kimura H, Iwai N, Ando S, et al. A prospective study of indications for mediastinoscopy in lung cancer with CT findings, tumor size, and tumor markers. Ann Thorac Surg 2003;75:1734–9.

[77] Riordain D, Buckley D, Aherne T. Mediastinoscopy as a predictor of resectability in patients with bronchogenic carcinoma. Ir J Med Sci 1991;160:291–2.

[78] Venissac N, Alifano M, Mouroux J. Video-assisted mediastinoscopy: experience from 240 consecutive cases. Ann Thorac Surg 2003;76(1):208–12.

[79] Herth FJ, Eberhardt R, Vilmann P, et al. Real-time endobronchial ultrasound guided transbronchial needle aspiration for sampling mediastinal lymph nodes. Thorax 2006;61(9):795–8.

[80] Yasufuku K, Chiyo M, Sekine Y, et al. Real-time endobronchial ultrasound-guided transbronchial needle aspiration of mediastinal and hilar lymph nodes. Chest 2004;126(1):122–8.

[81] Vilmann P, Krasnik M, Larsen SS, et al. Transesophageal endoscopic ultrasound-guided fine-needle aspiration (EUS-FNA) and endobronchial ultrasound-guided transbronchial needle aspiration (EBUS-TBNA) biopsy: a combined approach in the evaluation of mediastinal lesions. Endoscopy 2005;37:833–9.

[82] Yasufuku K, Nakajima T, Motoori K, et al. Comparison of endobronchial ultrasound, positron emission tomography, and CT for lymph node staging of lung cancer. Chest 2006;130:710–8.

[83] Vincent BD, El-Bayoumi E, Hoffman B, et al. Real-time endobronchial ultrasound guided transbronchial lymph node aspiration. Ann Thorac Surg 2008;85:224–30.

[84] Annema J, Veselic M, Rabe K. Analysis of subcarinal lymph nodes in (suspected) non-small-cell lung cancer after a negative transbronchial needle aspiration—what's next? Respiration 2004;71:630–4.

[85] Caddy G, Conron M, Wright G, et al. The accuracy of EUS-FNA in assessing mediastinal lymphadenopathy and staging patients with NSCLC. Eur Respir J 2005;25(3):410–5.

[86] Larsen SS, Vilmann P, Krasnik M, et al. Endoscopic ultrasound guided biopsy versus mediastinoscopy for analysis of paratracheal and subcarinal lymph nodes in lung cancer staging. Lung Cancer 2005; 48(1):85–92.

[87] Sawhney MS, Bakman Y, Holmstrom AM, et al. Impact of preoperative endoscopic ultrasound on non-small cell lung cancer staging. Chest 2007;132:916–21.

[88] Kramer H, van Putten JW, Post WJ, et al. Oesophageal endoscopic ultrasound with fine needle aspiration improves and simplifies the staging of lung cancer. Thorax 2004;59(7):596–601.

[89] Larsen SS, Krasnik M, Vilmann P, et al. Endoscopic ultrasound guided biopsy of mediastinal lesions has a major impact on patient management. Thorax 2002;57(2):98–103.

[90] Tournoy KG, Ryck FD, Vanwalleghem L, et al. The yield of endoscopic ultrasound in lung cancer staging: does lymph node size matter? J Thorac Oncol 2008;3:245–9.

[91] Cerfolio RJ, Bryant AS, Ojha B, et al. Improving the inaccuracies of clinical staging of patients with NSCLC: a prospective trial. Ann Thorac Surg 2005;80(4):1207–14.

[92] Eloubeidi M, Tamhane A. EUS-guided FNA of solid pancreatic masses: a learning curve with 300 consecutive procedures. Gastrointest Endosc 2005;61:700–8.

[93] Eloubeidi M, Tamhane A, Chen VE, et al. Endoscopic ultrasound-guided fine-needle aspiration in patients with non-small cell lung cancer and prior negative mediastinoscopy. Ann Thorac Surg 2005; 80:1231–9.

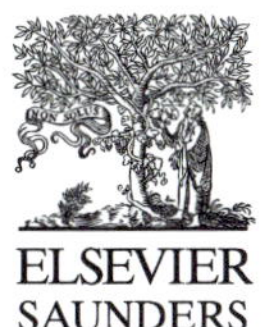
ELSEVIER
SAUNDERS

Thorac Surg Clin 18 (2008) 381–391

THORACIC SURGERY CLINICS

Intraoperative Staging and Surgical Management of Stage IIIA/N2 Non–Small Cell Lung Cancer

Igor Brichkov, MD, Steven M. Keller, MD*

Department of Cardiothoracic Surgery, Division of Thoracic Surgery, Albert Einstein College of Medicine, Montefiore Medical Center, 3400 Bainbridge Avenue – 5th floor, Bronx, NY 10467, USA

The treatment of patients with non–small-cell lung cancer (NSCLC) metastatic to the N2 lymph nodes disease remains controversial. All investigators agree, however, that the presence of tumor in the mediastinal lymph nodes represents advanced disease and is associated with an increased likelihood of death from NSCLC when compared with patients whose tumors are localized to the lung or have not spread beyond the N1 lymph nodes. The reported median and 5-year survival rate with N2 disease has a wide range and is probably related less to treatment than to the manner in which the N2 disease was documented. A careful reading of the pertinent literature spanning the last few decades demonstrates that the manner in which N2 disease was identified largely reflected institutional philosophy and was in turn influenced by available radiologic technology and an individual surgeon's interest and skill. These factors conspired to (unintentionally) create a host of N2 subcategories, among which are N2 found on posteroanterior chest radiograph, CT scan, positron emission tomographic scan, routine mediastinoscopy, intraoperative nodal sampling/dissection, intraoperative nodal sampling after a negative mediastinoscopy, and intraoperative nodal sampling after negative radiologic testing. Direct comparison of these disparate patient cohorts is difficult.

A categorization of postoperative N2 subgroups has been suggested by Detterbeck [1] that avoids the uncertainties associated with changing technology and reflects realistically clinical practice. He proposed four categories based on the time of discovery and the preoperative evaluation. (1) Incidental N2. A patient has had a thorough preoperative evaluation and intraoperative nodal sampling/dissection. N2 disease is documented postoperatively in the final pathology report. (2) Unsuspected N2. A patient has had a thorough preoperative evaluation and intraoperative nodal sampling/dissection. N2 disease is documented intraoperatively. (3) Ignored N2. A patient had suspicious N2 nodes noted on radiologic studies but did not have preoperative biopsy. N2 disease is documented intraoperatively or postoperatively. (4) Underappreciated N2. A patient is known to be at risk for N2 disease because of a central tumor or radiologic N1 involvement. N2 disease is documented intraoperatively or postoperatively. The categorization of preoperative N2 disease remains problematic.

Preoperative staging is not the focus of this article but deserves mention because it may influence intraoperative staging. Currently, before surgery, all patients should undergo CT and positron emission tomographic scans. Enlarged or avid mediastinal lymph nodes should be biopsied via mediastinoscopy, mediastinotomy, endobronchial ultrasound, or esophageal ultrasound. Extrathoracic sites of presumed metastases also require biopsy to ensure proper staging. A thorough history and physical examination remain an integral part of preoperative staging.

Intraoperative staging

The surgeon's responsibility extends beyond mere extirpation of the pulmonary tumor. In

* Corresponding author.
E-mail address: skeller@montefiore.org (S.M. Keller).

1547-4127/08/$ - see front matter
doi:10.1016/j.thorsurg.2008.08.003

thoracic.theclinics.com

addition to systematic lymph node sampling/dissection (*vide infra*), a thorough visual and tactile examination of the entire hemithorax is necessary to identify unanticipated intrathoracic disease processes that may or may not be related to the underlying malignancy. Biopsy is necessary to provide accurate pathologic TNM staging. The American Joint Commission on Cancer (AJCC)/Union Internationale Contre le Cancer (UICC) TNM definitions and stage groupings established in 2002 will be modified in 2009 [2–4]. These changes are based on analysis of data from 67,725 patients from 45 institutions in 20 countries on four continents who have NSCLC. Only those changes applicable to intraoperative staging will be described.

T descriptor

T1 tumors, which are smaller than 3 cm and surrounded by parenchyma, will be divided into T1a (<2 cm) and T1b (2–3 cm). T2 tumors, which are larger than 3 cm or of any size that involve the pleura, will be divided into T2a (3–5 cm) and T2b (5–7 cm). Tumors larger than 7 cm will be assigned to the T3 category. Most significantly, satellite nodules in the same lobe as the primary tumor, formerly T4, will be considered T3. Tumors in another ipsilateral lobe will be considered T4 rather than M1. Certain T4 tumors with regional spread (malignant pleural or pericardial effusions, pleural nodules) will be moved into the M1a category.

N descriptor

No changes in the currently accepted Mountain–Dresler lymph node level definitions [5] were recommended [3]. Grouping of nodal levels associated with similar prognoses into zones was proposed, however.

M descriptor

M1 metastases, which occur in another lobe of the ipsilateral lung or any metastases outside the hemithorax containing the primary tumor, will be divided into M1a and M1b. M1a will represent tumors with malignant pleural effusion, malignant pericardial effusions, or malignant pleural nodules. Patients with contralateral pulmonary metastases will be considered M1a.

Procedures for intraoperative nodal staging

Standardized definitions of the several techniques for intraoperative nodal assessment have been proposed but have not yet been universally accepted [6]. Selected lymph node biopsy involves biopsy of one or more suspicious nodes discovered at the time of exploration. The only role of this technique is to obtain lymph nodes not accessible by preoperative invasive staging procedures, and it serves to rule in N2 disease in patients deemed unresectable. Sampling involves removal of one or more lymph nodes deemed to be suspicious by preoperative imaging or intraoperative assessment. Systematic sampling involves removal of one or more lymph nodes at several predetermined mediastinal levels. This approach is not a full mediastinal lymph node dissection but seeks to address the nodal status of a representative sample of the mediastinal lymph nodes.

Systematic lymph node dissection (SLND) is the more classically described mediastinal lymph node dissection characterized by the complete removal of all mediastinal lymph node–baring tissue from at least three nodal levels. Also included is the removal of lobar and hilar nodes. All nodal levels are removed, labeled, and sent separately for histologic analysis. Lobe-specific systematic lymph node dissection is a modification of SLND, in which only the nodal stations that correspond to sites that have a high likelihood of containing metastasis are excised. The most invasive procedure along the spectrum of mediastinal nodal assessment is the extended lymph node dissection. Proposed by Watanabe [7] and popularized by Hata [8], this radical lymph node dissection is performed through a sternotomy with a cervical collar extension incision. It involves the complete removal of all nodal tissue at all bilateral mediastinal levels and nodes in the scalene stations and low cervical nodal drainage basins. The increased morbidity of performing a sternotomy and a thoracotomy and the increased risk of phrenic and recurrent laryngeal nerve injuries have prevented dissemination of this technique.

Comparison of nodal assessment techniques

Gaer and colleagues [9] compared intraoperative assessment by the surgeon to histopathologic examination of the resected lymph nodes in 95 patients. All patients underwent SLND after pulmonary resection for NSCLC. Samples taken from

287 nodal levels were examined by the surgeon and submitted for microscopic examination. They found that assessment by the surgeon had a sensitivity of only 71% and a positive predictive value of only 64%. Haiderer [10] found that 4.1% of patients with normal appearing lymph nodes had evidence of metastasis. Bollen [11] reported that N2 disease was 2.1 times (95% confidence interval 1.04–4.2) more likely to be detected in patients who underwent either systematic sampling or SLND as compared with selective sampling. These results can be explained by the fact that micrometastases may not be palpable to the surgeon intraoperatively and suggest that neither selected lymph node biopsy nor selective sampling are sensitive enough techniques to provide an adequate intraoperative assessment of N2 status.

Graham [12] demonstrated that N2 disease could be documented in 20% of patients with preoperatively negative radiographic and mediastinoscopic evaluations by performing SLND during intraoperative nodal staging. The answer to whether systematic sampling or a more extensive lymph node dissection is necessary to adequately stage the mediastinum has been found in several recent studies. Izbicki [13] prospectively compared systematic sampling to SLND (all levels) and found that the proportion of patients in whom N2 disease was identified intraoperatively was similar for both techniques. In retrospective studies, Keller [14] and Takizawa [15] reported similar results. Although the two techniques seem to be equally efficacious for staging, SLND is more likely to document the presence of N2 disease at multiple lymph node levels [13,14]. Although this information does not alter TNM stage, a more complete assessment of extent of disease is obtained.

Is the technique used to assess the mediastinal lymph nodes crucial for accurate staging or are the number of lymph nodes sampled the determining factor? Using Surveillance, Epidemiology and End Results (SEER) database, Ludwig and colleagues [16] analyzed the survival of 15,789 patients who underwent resection of pathologic stage I NSCLC between 1990 and 2000. The number of lymph nodes contained in the pathologic specimen was grouped: 1 to 4, 5 to 8, 9 to 12, and 13 to 16. The lymph nodes were not exclusively mediastinal. A survival benefit was seen when 5 or more nodes were removed and continued incrementally as the number of lymph nodes removed increased. The authors thought the results reflected stage migration and concluded that removal of 10 to 11 lymph nodes ensured accurate staging. Other investigators suggested, however, that removal of 6 total nodes (at least three mediastinal nodes) [17] or 10 nodes [18] (at least two mediastinal levels) was associated with improved survival for patients with resected stage I NSCLC.

The European Society of Thoracic Surgery recommends SLND for all patients undergoing resection for NSCLC [6]. For right lung tumors, levels 2 to 4 and levels 7 to 9 should be excised in an en-bloc fashion. For left lung cancers, a minimum of levels 4 to 6 and levels 7 to 9 should be removed. Access to the higher left paratracheal nodes may be obtained by dividing the ligamentum arteriosum. The European Society of Thoracic Surgery guidelines recognize a lobar-specific dissection for peripheral T1 squamous tumors.

Technique of systematic lymph node dissection

Systematic lymph node dissection is easily accomplished via posterolateral or muscle-sparing thoracotomy using split-lung ventilation and typically follows the pulmonary resection. SLND also can be performed as part of a video-assisted thoracoscopic (VATS) lobectomy, although the level 7 (subcarinal) lymph nodes may be difficult to access via the left chest. Lymph nodes harvested from the different levels must be labeled appropriately (including right or left when appropriate) and sent from the operating room as carefully marked separate specimens. Improper identification of the specimens can negate the value of the most meticulous of lymph node dissections and complicates postoperative treatment plans.

Right hemithorax

Entry into the chest through the fourth or fifth interspace provides access to the necessary lymph node levels. The superior mediastinum, encompassed by the superior vena cava, trachea, and azygous vein, is exposed by retracting the lung caudally and posteriorly (Fig. 1). The phrenic nerve can be identified on the lateral aspect of the superior vena cava. The vagus nerve can be visualized through the unopened pleura as it traverses the superior mediastinum craniocaudally. The mediastinal pleura, cephalad to the azygous vein and between the trachea and superior vena cava, is grasped with forceps and incised to the

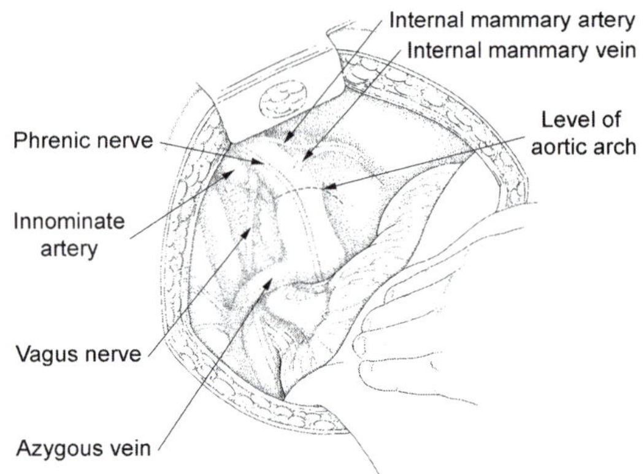

Fig. 1. Exposure of right superior mediastinum with mediastinal pleura intact. (*Courtesy of* S. Keller, MD, Bronx, NY.)

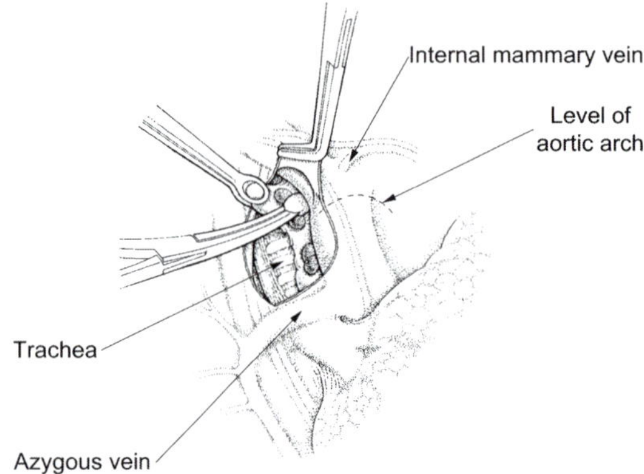

Fig. 2. The internal mammary vein drains into the approximate juncture between the right and left innominate veins as they combine to form the superior vena cava. It is a reliable structure with which to differentiate the division between level 2 and level 4 lymph nodes. The dashed line represents the aortic arch. (*Courtesy of* S. Keller, MD, Bronx, NY.)

level of the innominate artery. The pleural edge overlying the trachea is retracted posteriorly, and the mediastinal fat pad is bluntly dissected off the anterolateral aspect of the trachea using a peanut sponge on a clamp. Similarly, the pleural edge over the superior vena cava is retracted anteriorly, and the mediastinal fat pad is dissected from the junction of the superior vena cava and the azygous vein to the level of the innominate artery. A small vein is frequently encountered draining into the superior vena cava posterolaterally and should be ligated or clipped to avoid unnecessary bleeding. Nonmagnetic clips should be used to occlude all small blood vessels and lymphatics seen entering the mediastinal fat pad in an attempt to prevent prolonged postoperative chest drainage and minimize blood loss.

Right level 2 lymph nodes are located between the cephalad border of the innominate vein and the cephalad border of the aortic arch (Fig. 2). Lymph nodes lying between the cephalad border of the aortic arch and the cephalad border of the azygous vein (Fig. 3) are excised and labeled as right level 4 superior. Next, the azygous vein is elevated with a vein retractor. Lymph nodes located between the cephalad border of the azygous vein and the origin of the right upper lobe bronchus (Fig. 4) are removed and labeled as right level 4 inferior. During this part of the dissection, care must be taken not to injure the pulmonary artery, superior vena cava, or phrenic nerve.

Dissection between the esophagus and membranous portion of the trachea at a level cephalad to the azygous vein reveals the right level 3 posterior nodes. Right level 3 anterior nodes are found anterior and medial to the superior vena cava at the insertion of the azygous vein. Right level 10 nodes are seen along the anterior border of the bronchus intermedius distal to the pleural reflection and are exposed by retracting the lung posteriorly and the pulmonary artery anteriorly (Fig. 5). Right level 11 lymph nodes are found in the sump of Borrie between the lobar bronchi. Exposure is provided by posterior retraction of the lung. Right level 12 lymph nodes are situated at the distal aspect of the lobar bronchi and are resected with the specimen (Fig. 6). Clips should

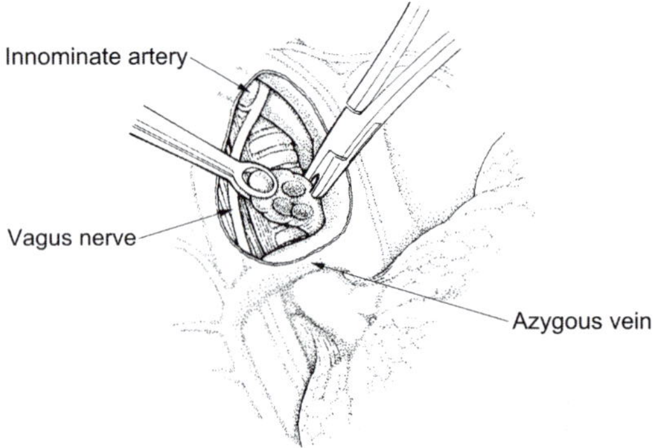

Fig. 3. The lymphadenectomy may be extended to the contralateral lymph node levels (not shown). Care must be taken not to injure the left recurrent laryngeal nerve, which is found in the tracheoesophageal groove. (*Courtesy of* S. Keller, MD, Bronx, NY.)

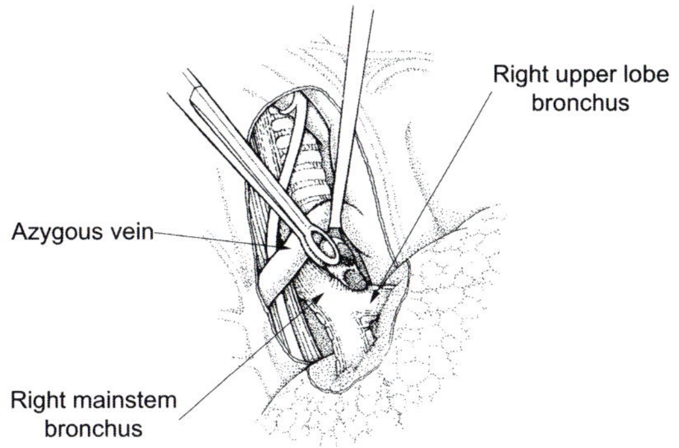

Fig. 4. Division of the azygous vein is rarely necessary. (*Courtesy of* S. Keller, MD, Bronx, NY.)

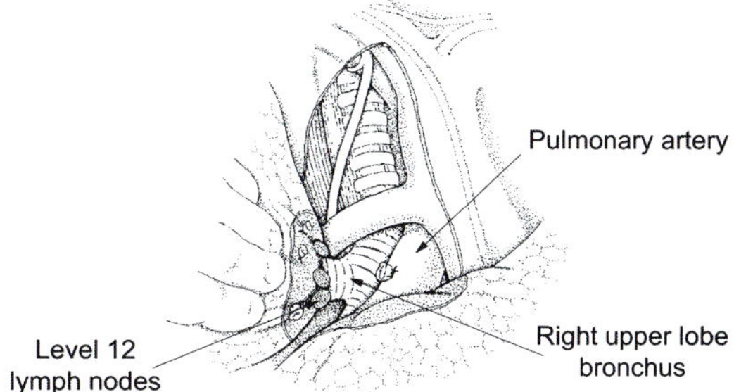

Fig. 6. A peanut is used to dissect the level 12 lymph nodes and include them with the specimen. Cautery is used to transect soft tissue, because a clip may interfere with application of a stapling device. (*Courtesy of* S. Keller, MD, Bronx, NY.)

be avoided in this area if a stapling device is to be used for division of the bronchus.

The level 7 nodes are exposed by retracting the lung anteriorly and opening the mediastinal pleura. The pleural edge overlying the esophagus is grasped and retracted posteriorly with the esophagus. A malleable retractor or sponge stick may be used to retract and protect the esophagus (Fig. 7). A ring clamp is used to grasp and elevate the subcarinal fat pad. Attachments to the right and left mainstem bronchi are divided. An arterial vessel entering the subcarinal fat pad from behind the carina is frequently encountered and should be ligated. The right level 9 lymph nodes are found in the inferior pulmonary ligament and are resected using clips or cautery. Right level 8 nodes may or may not be present. Bleeding from the SLND is minimal and can be controlled with topical hemostatic agents and direct pressure. Accumulation of clear fluid may indicate an unsecured lymphatic channel. To minimize the possibility of a postoperative chylothorax, the source should be identified and ligated.

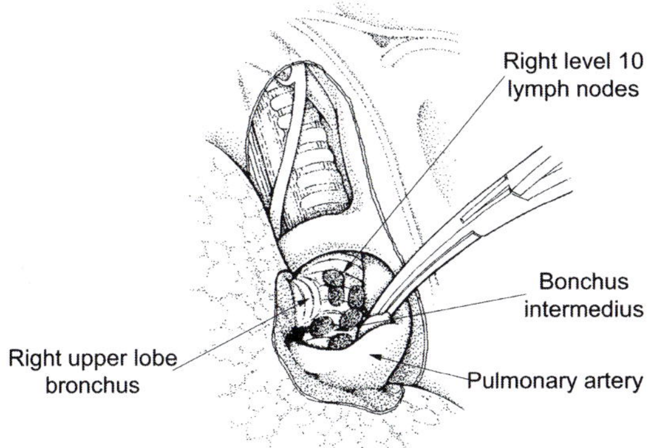

Fig. 5. Exposure of the level 10 lymph nodes is accomplished by retracting the pulmonary artery anteriorly. (*Courtesy of* S. Keller, MD, Bronx, NY.)

Left hemithorax

Access to the lymph node levels is achieved by entering the pleural cavity in the fifth or sixth interspace. The lung is retracted caudally to expose the aortopulmonary window. The phrenic and vagus nerves are identified running parallel and traversing the mediastinum craniocaudally. The pleura overlying the aortopulmonary window is elevated and incised in a cephalad direction midway between and parallel to the phrenic and vagus nerves. The ligamentum arteriosum is easily identified by palpation. The pleural edge nearest to the phrenic nerve is retracted anteriorly. Level 6 lymph nodes are located in the fat pad anterior to the ligamentum arteriosum and are swept posteriorly to avoid injury to the phrenic nerve. Level 5 lymph nodes are found posterior to the ligamentum arteriosum. Injury to the nearby recurrent

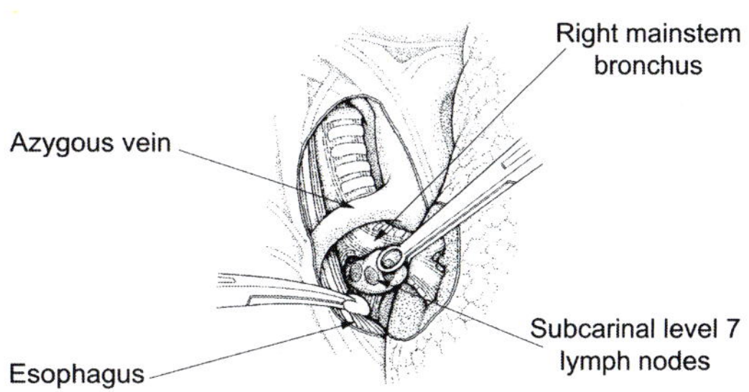

Fig. 7. The esophagus and membranous portion of the bronchus must not be injured when applying clips. (*Courtesy of* S. Keller, MD, Bronx, NY.)

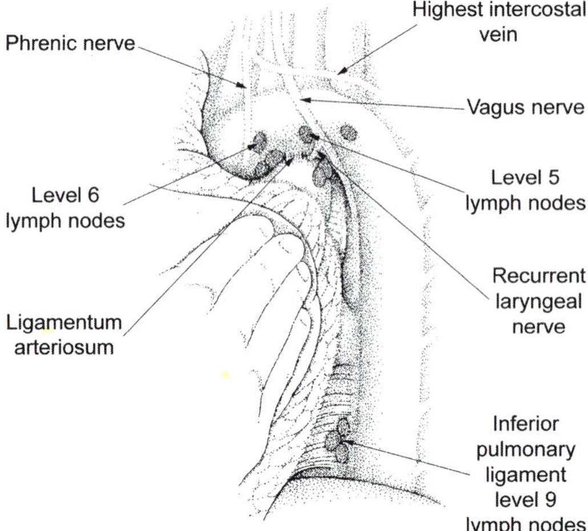

Fig. 8. The left superior mediastinum before opening the mediastinal pleura. Exposure of level 2 or 4 lymph nodes would require mobilization of the aortic arch. (*Courtesy of* S. Keller, MD, Bronx, NY.)

laryngeal nerve, which enters the mediastinum posterior to the ligamentum arteriosum, is avoided by using blunt dissection (Fig. 8). Clips rather than cautery should be used for hemostasis.

Level 7 nodes are exposed by retracting the lung anteriorly and extending the pleural incision in a caudal direction just anterior to the aorta. The aorta is retracted posteriorly and the left mainstem bronchus is identified inferomedial to the pulmonary artery (Fig. 9). The subcarinal fat pad is grasped with a ring forceps. Care must be taken to avoid injuring the esophagus, because it lies just medial to the aorta and may not be readily apparent when beginning the subcarinal nodal dissection. Attachments to the right and left mainstem bronchi are clipped. Vessels entering the subcarinal fat pad must be ligated. Left level 11 nodes are located distal to the pleural reflection in the area between the lobar bronchi and are exposed by retracting the pulmonary artery posteriorly. Care must be taken to avoid injuring the interlobar pulmonary artery. Left level 12 nodes are situated along the distal aspect of the lobar bronchus and are usually removed with the specimen (Fig. 10). Left level 9 lymph nodes can be identified in the inferior pulmonary ligament and are removed with clips or cautery. Left level 8 lymph nodes may be present and are identified along the distal esophagus.

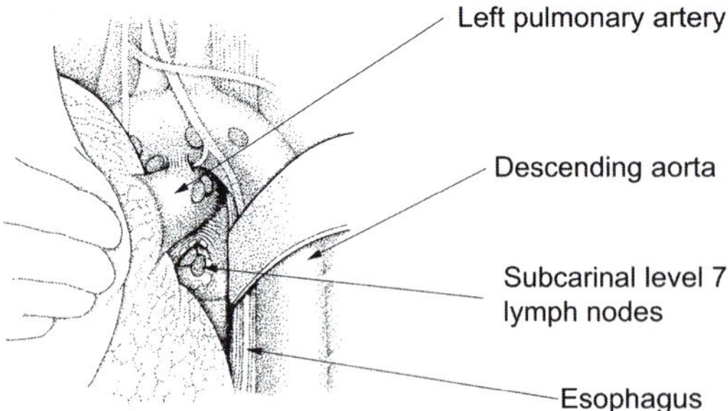

Fig. 9. The subcarinal lymph nodes are more difficult to expose in the left hemithorax than in the right hemithorax. A malleable retractor is used to retract the aorta and esophagus posteriorly. (*Courtesy of* S. Keller, MD, Bronx, NY.)

Thoracoscopy and nodal staging

During the past decade, several investigators have compared VATS lobectomy to open lobectomy (standard or muscle sparing) for the surgical management of NSCLC. Reported advantages of the VATS approach include smaller incisions, decreased blood loss, decreased postoperative pain, improved postoperative immunologic and pulmonary function, decreased length of stay, and decreased hospital costs. Although an anatomic pulmonary resection can be accomplished readily via VATS, the ability to perform an SLND has been questioned.

In order to compare the thoroughness of lymph node dissection, Sugi [19] prospectively randomized 100 consecutive patients with clinical stage I NSCLC to either VATS lobectomy or open thoracotomy. Fifty patients were assigned to each arm. The number of lymph nodes harvested did not differ, with a mean of 8 hilar and 13 mediastinal lymph nodes removed in both

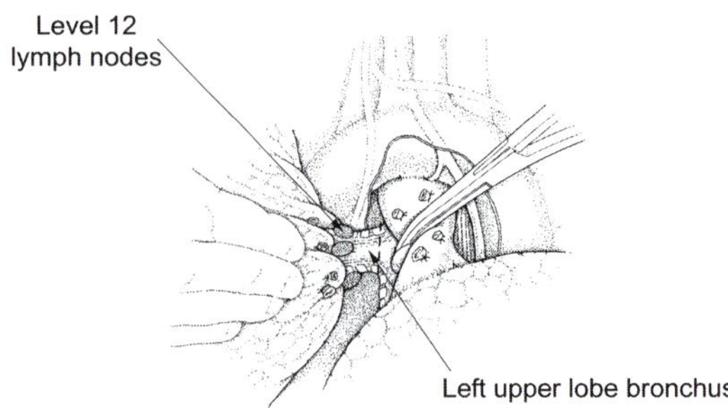

Fig. 10. As the soft tissue is cleared to permit application of the stapling device, the nodes are pushed distally with a peanut. (*Courtesy of* S. Keller, MD, Bronx, NY.)

groups. Actuarial 5-year survival rates were 85% and 90% for the open and VATS groups, respectively. Locoregional recurrence occurred in 19% and 10% for the open and VATS groups, respectively. The differences were not statistically significant. Sagawa prospectively [20] assessed the adequacy of mediastinal lymph node dissection during a VATS lobectomy in 35 patients with clinical stage I NSCLC. After thoracoscopic lymph node dissection, a different surgeon performed a thoracotomy to assess the completeness of the lymph node dissection. In the right chest, an average of 40.3 lymph nodes were harvested via VATS and an additional 1.2 (range 0–6) were removed by thoracotomy. In the left hemithorax, an average of 37.1 lymph nodes were removed via VATS and an additional 1.2 (range 0–4) were obtained by thoracotomy.

Morbidity associated with lymph node dissection

Bollen [11] found no difference in the intraoperative blood loss or transfusion requirements among patients with NSCLC who underwent pulmonary resection and had no sampling, systematic sampling, or SLND. There was increased chest tube drainage in patients who underwent systematic sampling or SLND, however. Recurrent laryngeal nerve injury was reported in three (5%) patients, and chylothorax was reported in two patients who underwent SLND. Bronchopleural fistulas were reported in two patients who did not undergo any lymph node dissection. Hata [8] reported two recurrent laryngeal nerve paralyses and one phrenic injury among 55 patients who underwent extended mediastinal lymph node dissection.

In a prospective randomized trial of 182 patients who underwent either systematic sampling or SLND, Izbicki [21] found no difference in blood loss, mortality, need for reoperation, chest tube drainage, and length of stay between the two groups. One chylothorax occurred in each group. Recurrent laryngeal nerve injury was reported in 6 patients who underwent systematic sampling and 5 patients who underwent SLND. SLND extended the procedure by 20 minutes.

In an unplanned analysis of a phase III adjuvant therapy trial (n = 373), Keller [14] found no significant difference in blood loss, transfusion requirement, and duration of operation between patients who underwent either systematic sampling or SLND. These results were confirmed by the ACOSOG Z0030 [22] trial, in which patients who underwent SLND as compared with systematic sampling had a longer median operative time of 15 minutes and 121 mL of increased chest tube drainage. These differences were statistically significant but clinically insignificant.

Survival advantage of lymph node dissection

Several authors have suggested that SLND is associated with improved survival. This survival advantage may be caused by the eradication of truly localized metastatic disease. Izbicki [23] documented that patients undergoing SLND were found to have improved overall survival rates (70% vs. 38%) and disease-free survival rates (59% vs. 21%) as compared with systematic sampling when the nodal disease burden was N1 or single node N2. Keller [14] reported a statistically significant survival benefit in patients with right lung tumors undergoing SLND. In a prospective randomized trial of 532 patients, Wu found a 48% versus 37% survival benefit of SLND as compared with systematic sampling [24]. This survival benefit was also seen when patients were compared by stage. A meta-analysis including 997 patients also showed a significant survival benefit to SLND when compared with systematic sampling [25]. Other authors, however, have not identified any survival benefit [19,26]. The prospective randomized multicenter American College of Surgeons Oncology Group (ACOSOG) Z0030 trial should provide a more definitive answer to the question of improved survival following SLND for NSCLC once long-term survival data become available.

Newer mediastinal lymph node staging techniques

The importance of thoroughly staging the mediastinum in patients who have NSCLC has given rise to two new techniques of mediastinal lymphadenectomy. Video-assisted mediastinal lymphadenectomy evolved from the notion that conventional mediastinoscopy is limited to biopsy of lymph node levels 2, 4, and 7. By improving visualization of the superior mediastinum and expanding the fields of access to the anterior mediastinum using the expanding twin-bladed Linder-Dahan video-mediastinoscope, Bitte [27,28] was able to perform a SLND through a small transverse cervical incision. Video-assisted mediastinal lymphadenectomy was performed on

144 patients with NSCLC and results compared with intraoperative SLND performed during pulmonary resection on the same patients. Video-assisted mediastinal lymphadenectomy showed a sensitivity of 100% and a specificity of 93.75%. The median operative time was 54 minutes. Complications occurred in 4% of patients: five recurrent nerve injuries, one arterial injury, and two venous injuries. There was no mortality. Combining video-assisted mediastinal lymphadenectomy with a VATS lobectomy may provide the ability to perform a true SLND and anatomic pulmonary resection with minimally invasive procedures.

Transcervical extended mediastinal lymphadenectomy resulted from combining the extended mediastinal lymphadenectomy with the surgical approach for transcervical thymectomy. Using a cervical collar incision and retracting the upper sternum anteriorly, Kuzdal [29] identified and excised lymph nodes at levels 1 to 8 bilaterally. Sensitivity and specificity rates were 90% and 100%, respectively. Mean operative time was 191 minutes (range 120–350 minutes). Complications were documented in 13% of patients: four recurrent nerve injuries and two pneumothoraces. No patients died. Diagnostic yield was similar to that of the extended mediastinal lymph node dissection described by Hata [8]. The disadvantages of transcervical extended mediastinal lymphadenectomy are increased operative time, potential morbidity of an extended bilateral lymphadenectomy, and lack of justification for such an extensive dissection.

Surgical management of stage IIIa/N2 non–small-cell lung cancer

Preoperatively identified N2 disease

Most thoracic oncologists and thoracic surgeons would agree that N2 disease that presents as multiple large lymph nodes located at multiple nodal levels is unlikely to ever become resectable and is best treated with definitive concurrent radiotherapy and chemotherapy. These same physicians would passionately debate the role of surgery for patients with potentially removable N2 disease, however. If surgery is contemplated, all would agree that some neoadjuvant therapy is indicated. Every neoadjuvant phase II and most neoadjuvant phase III trials have assumed that surgery must play a role and have asked chemotherapy or radiotherapy questions. Only two randomized prospective phase III trials have questioned the role of surgery in patients with potentially resectable N2 disease.

The European Organization for Research and Treatment of Cancer-Lung Cancer Group treated 579 patients with pathologically demonstrated N2 disease with induction chemotherapy [30]. Sixty-one percent responded and were eligible for randomization between surgery and radiotherapy. Median and 5-year survivals were 16.4 months versus 17.5 months and 15.7% versus 14%, respectively. Neither difference was statistically significant. The authors concluded that radiotherapy was the preferred local therapy after induction chemotherapy. The Radiation Therapy Oncology Group treated 429 patients with histologically documented N2 disease with concurrent chemotherapy and radiotherapy [31]. Responders were randomized to either surgery or additional radiotherapy. Median and 5-year survival figures were 23.6 months and 27.2% versus 22.2 months and 20.3%, respectively. Once again, no statistical difference was found. Unplanned subgroup analyses in both studies suggested that patients whose disease could be removed with a lobectomy had improved survival when compared with patients who required pneumonectomy.

Should these results of these two large trials interdict surgery for all patients with preoperatively identified N2 disease? Is there a subgroup of patients with preoperatively identified minimal N2 disease (eg, single nodal level, microscopic only) who will benefit from surgery? If so, should the neoadjuvant therapy consist of radiotherapy and chemotherapy? The answers to these questions are currently unknown. Future phase III trials will address these important questions.

Postoperatively identified N2 disease

Patients with resected N2 disease should be offered cisplatin-based adjuvant chemotherapy. The Adjuvant Navalbine International Trialist Association phase III trial compared adjuvant navelbine and cisplatin to observation in patients who had undergone resection of stages Ib-IIIa NSCLC [32]. For the subgroup of patients with N2 disease (n = 224), the investigators demonstrated a statistically significant absolute 5-year survival benefit of 21% (40% vs. 19%) in favor of the treatment arm. Similarly, the International Adjuvant Lung Cancer Trial Cooperative Group phase III trial demonstrated a survival benefit for the cohort of patients (n = 479) with resected N2 disease who received cisplatin-based chemotherapy [33]. Meta-analyses such as that by the Lung Adjuvant Cisplatin Evaluation Collaborative Group confirmed the survival benefits of adjuvant cisplatin-based chemotherapy for patients with resected stages II and IIIa NSCLC. Although patients with N2 disease were not analyzed separately, it is reasonable to assume that most patients in the stage IIIa group had metastases to the mediastinal lymph nodes [34].

The benefit of postoperative radiotherapy (PORT) in patients with resected N2 disease remains unproven. Few randomized prospective trials are available to provide guidance. A recent phase III trial containing 190 patients with N2 disease showed no benefit for PORT [35]. Lally and colleagues [36] reviewed the SEER data of 7465 patients with stages II and IIIa NSCLC who had undergone complete resection. N2 disease was present in 1987 patients, 62% of whom received PORT. The 5-year survival rate was 27% in patients who had received PORT versus 20% in patients who had not ($P = .0036$). Two meta-analyses have shown no survival benefit for PORT, however. The PORT Meta-analysis Trialists Group reviewed the individual data of 2128 patients from nine randomized trials [37]. A detrimental affect of PORT was reported for patients with stages I and II. The number of patients with N2 disease was not reported, although 808 patients were classified as stage IIIa. Most of these patients likely had N2 disease. Subgroup analyses of patients with either stage IIIa or N2 disease did not reveal an adverse affect of PORT, but neither was a benefit found. An updated meta-analysis by the same group once again demonstrated no survival benefit for patients with resected N2 disease (n = 550) who received PORT [38]. A European phase III trial of PORT (Lung Adjuvant Radiotherapy Trial) in patients with resected N2 disease is currently accruing patients.

Intraoperatively identified N2 disease

The subgroup with the least data to guide clinical practice consists of patients in whom N2 disease is discovered intraoperatively. Ferguson [39] performed an interesting and thoughtful cost-effectiveness analysis that addressed the question of what should be done if N2 disease is discovered during surgery. Based on a meta-analysis of 1046 patients without clinical evidence of N2 disease who underwent resection and 775 patients who had N2 identified before surgery and were treated with some form of neoadjuvant therapy, he concluded that if N2 disease is identified in the operating room, the planned resection should be aborted and the patient treated with chemotherapy and radiotherapy. Depending on the response to neoadjuvant therapy, the patient might or might not return to the operating at some future date. Some of the essential model assumptions, although reasonable at the time of publication, are not supported by more recent data.

Detterbeck [1] recently published a thorough review of this topic, one that is worth reading in detail. Data pooled from numerous studies were analyzed to determine negative and positive prognostic factors associated with resection of N2 disease. Favorable elements included T1-2 tumors, metastases to a single nodal level, preoperative clinical N0-1 disease, and upper lobe tumors metastatic only to regional nodes (right to level 4, left to level 5). Unfavorable influences included multilevel N2 disease, T3-4 tumors, and subcarinal metastases. These results were combined with other components, such as the ability to administer neoadjuvant or adjuvant therapies and the morbidity/mortality associated with surgery, to determine if surgery should proceed once intraoperative N2 disease is discovered. He concluded that if N2 disease is identified in the operating room, every effort (commensurate with the patient's ability to tolerate the operation) should be made to remove the primary tumor and all the involved lymph nodes.

Summary

Staging of the mediastinum is an integral component of the operative treatment of NSCLC. Systematic sampling and systematic lymph node dissection provide similar and accurate staging information. Systematic lymph node dissection is more likely to identify multiple levels of N2 disease, however, and may be associated with improved survival. During surgery for a right lung cancer, at least mediastinal lymph node levels 4 should be sampled or dissected. When removing a left lung cancer, at least nodal levels 5 and 7 should be assessed. Although every effort should be made to identify N2 disease before surgery, if intraoperative metastases to mediastinal lymph nodes are discovered, the planned operation should proceed. Cisplatin-based adjuvant chemotherapy has moderate but proven survival benefit after resection of N2 disease. The role of PORT remains uncertain.

References

[1] Detterbeck F. What to do with "surprise" N2? Intraoperative management of patients with non-small cell lung cancer. J Thorac Oncol 2008;3:289–302.

[2] Rami-Porta R, Ball D, Crowley J, et al. The IASLC lung cancer staging project: proposals for the revision of the T descriptors in the forthcoming (seventh) edition of the TNM classification for lung cancer. J Thorac Oncol 2007;2:593–602.

[3] Rusch VW, Crowler J, Giroux DJ, et al. The IASLC lung cancer staging project: proposals for the revision of the N descriptors in the forthcoming seventh edition of the TNM classification for lung cancer. J Thorac Oncol 2007;2:603–12.

[4] Goldstraw P, Crowley J, Chansky K, et al. The IASLC lung cancer staging project: proposals for the revision of the TNM stage groupings in the forthcoming (seventh) edition of the TNM classification for lung cancer. J Thorac Oncol 2007;2:706–14.

[5] Mountain CF, Dresler CM. Regional lymph node classification for lung cancer staging. Chest 1997; 111:1718–23.

[6] Lardinois D, De Leyn P, Van Schil P, et al. ESTS guidelines for intraoperative lymph node staging in non-small cell lung cancer. Eur J Cardiothorac Surg 2006;30:787–92.

[7] Watanabe Y, Shimizu J, Oda M, et al. Improved survival in left non-small-cell N2 lung cancer after more extensive operative procedure. Thorac Cardiovasc Surg 1991;39:89–94.

[8] Hata E, Miyamoto H, Tanaka M, et al. Superradical operation for lung cancer: bilateral mediastinal dissection (BMD) with or without cervical dissection (CD). Lung Cancer 1994;11(Suppl 2):41–6.

[9] Gaer JA, Goldstraw P. Intraoperative assessment of nodal staging at thoracotomy for carcinoma of the bronchus. Eur J Cardiothorac Surg 1990;4:207–10.

[10] Haiderer O, Wustinger E, Lexer G, et al. [Mediastinal lymphadenectomy: anatomical basis and its surgical relevance in central bronchus carcinoma]. Wien Med Wochenschr 1990;140:422–6 [in German].

[11] Bollen EC, van Duin CJ, Theunissen PH, et al. Mediastinal lymph node dissection in resected lung cancer: morbidity and accuracy of staging. Ann Thorac Surg 1993;55:961–6.

[12] Graham ANJ, Chan KJ, Pastorino U, et al. Systematic nodal dissection in the intrathoracic staging of patients with non-small cell lung cancer. J Thorac Cardiovasc Surg 1999;117:246–51.

[13] Izbicki JR, Passlick B, Karg O, et al. Impact of radical systematic mediastinal lymphadenectomy on tumor staging in lung cancer. Ann Thorac Surg 1995; 59:209–14.

[14] Keller SM, Adak S, Wagner H, et al. Mediastinal lymph node dissection improves survival in patients with stages II and IIIa non-small cell lung cancer. Eastern Cooperative Oncology Group. Ann Thorac Surg 2000;70:358–65.

[15] Takizawa H, Kondo K, Matsuoka H, et al. Effect of mediastinal lymph nodes sampling in patients with clinical stage I non-small cell lung cancer. J Med Invest 2008;55:37–43.

[16] Ludwig MS, Goodman M, Miller DL, et al. Postoperative survival and the number of lymph nodes sampled during resection of node-negative non-small cell lung cancer. Chest 2005;128:1545–50.

[17] Gajra A, Newman N, Gamble GP, et al. Effect of number of lymph nodes sampled on outcome in patients with stage I non-small-cell lung cancer. J Clin Oncol 2003;21:1029–34.

[18] Doddoli C, Aragon A, Berlesi F, et al. Does the extent of lymph node dissection influence outcome in patients with stage I non-small-cell lung cancer? Eur J Cardiothorac Surg. 2005;27:680–5.

[19] Sugi K, Nawata K, Fujita N, et al. Systematic lymph node dissection for clinically diagnosed peripheral non-small-cell lung cancer less than 2 cm in diameter. World J Surg 1998;22:290–4.

[20] Sagawa M, Sato M, Sakurada A, et al. A prospective trial of systematic nodal dissection for lung cancer by video-assisted thoracic surgery: can it be perfect? Ann Thorac Surg 2002;73:900–4.

[21] Izbicki JR, Thetter O, Habekost M, et al. Radical systematic mediastinal lymphadenectomy in non-small cell lung cancer: a randomized controlled trial. Br J Surg 1994;81:229–35.

[22] Allen MS, Darling G, Pechet T, et al. Morbidity and mortality of major pulmonary resections in patients with early stage lung cancer: initial results of the randomized, prospective ACOSOG Z0030 trial. Ann Thorac Surg 2006;81:1013–9.

[23] Izbicki JR, Passlick B, Pantel K, et al. Effectiveness of radical systematic mediastinal lymphadenectomy in patients with resectable non-small cell lung cancer: results of a prospective randomized trial. Ann Surg 1998;227:138–44.

[24] Wu Y, Huang ZF, Wang SY, et al. A randomized trial of systematic nodal dissection in resectable non-small cell lung cancer. Lung Cancer 2002;36: 1–6.

[25] Manser R, Wright G, Hart D, et al. Surgery for early stage non-small cell lung cancer. Cochrane Database of Systematic Reviews 2005;(1):CD004699. doi:10.1002/14651858.CD004699.pub2.

[26] Lardinois D, Suter H, Hakki H, et al. Morbidity, survival, and site of recurrence after mediastinal lymph node dissection versus systematic sampling after complete resection for non-small cell lung cancer. Ann Thorac Surg 2005;80: 268–74.

[27] Witte B, Wolf M, Huertgen M, et al. Video-assisted mediastinoscopic surgery: clinical feasibility and accuracy of mediastinal lymph node staging. Ann Thorac Surg 2006;82:1821–7.

[28] Witte B, Hurtgen M. Video-assisted mediastinoscopic lymphadenectomy (VAMLA). J Thorac Oncol 2007;2:367–9.

[29] Kuzdal J, Zielinski M, Papla B, et al. Transcervical extended mediastinal lymphadenectomy: the new operative technique and early results in lung cancer staging. Eur J Cardiothorac Surg 2005;27:384–90.

[30] van Meerbeeck JP, Kramer GW, Van Schil PE, et al. Randomized controlled trial of resection versus radiotherapy after induction chemotherapy in stage IIIA-N2 non–small-cell lung cancer. J Natl Cancer Inst 2007;99:442–50.

[31] Albain KS, Swann RS, Rusch VR, et al. Phase III study of concurrent chemotherapy and radiotherapy (CT/RT) vs CT/RT followed by surgical resection for stage IIIA(pN2) non-small cell lung cancer (NSCLC): outcomes update of North American Intergroup 0139 (RTOG 9309). J Clin Oncol 2005; 23(16s):624s [abstract 7014].

[32] Douillard JY, Rosell R, De Lena M, et al. Adjuvant vinorelbine plus cisplatin versus observation in patients with completely resected stage IB–IIIA non-small cell lung cancer (Adjuvant Navelbine International Trialist Association [ANITA]): a randomised controlled trial. Lancet Oncol 2006;7:719–27.

[33] The International Adjuvant Lung Cancer Trial Collaborative Group. Cisplatin-based adjuvant chemotherapy in patients with completely resected non-small-cell lung cancer. N Engl J Med 2004;350:351–60.

[34] Pignon JP, Tribodet H, Scagliotti GV, et al. Lung adjuvant cisplatin evaluation: a pooled analysis by the LACE Collaborative Group. J Clin Oncol 2008;26:[epub].

[35] Dautzenberg B, Arriagada R, Chammard AB, et al. A controlled study of postoperative radiotherapy for patients with completely resected nonsmall cell lung carcinoma. Cancer 1999;86:265–73.

[36] Lally BE, Zelterman D, Colasanto JM, et al. Postoperative radiotherapy for stage II or III non-small cell lung cancer using surveillance, epidemiology, and end results database. J Clin Oncol 2006;24: 2998–3006.

[37] PORT Meta-analysis Trialists Group. Postoperative radiotherapy in non-small-cell lung cancer: systematic review and meta-analysis of individual patient data from nine randomised controlled trials. Lancet 1998;352:257–63.

[38] PORT Meta-analysis Trialists Group. Postoperative radiotherapy for non-small cell lung cancer. Cochrane Database Syst Rev 2005;(2):CD002142.

[39] Ferguson MK. Optimal management when unsuspected N2 nodal disease is identified during thoracotomy for lung cancer: cost-effectiveness analysis. J Thorac Cardiovasc Surg 2003;126: 1935–42.

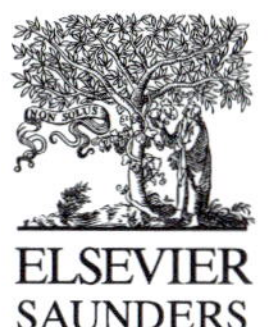

ELSEVIER
SAUNDERS

Thorac Surg Clin 18 (2008) 393–401

THORACIC
SURGERY
CLINICS

Definitive Chemoradiotherapy for Non–Small Cell Lung Cancer with N2 Disease

Shilpen Patel, MD[a,*], Rachel E. Sanborn, MD[b], Charles R. Thomas, Jr., MD[c]

[a]Department of Radiation Oncology, Fred Hutchinson Cancer Research Center, University of Washington, 1959 NE Pacific Street, Box 356043, Seattle, WA 98195, USA
[b]Providence Portland Medical Center, Portland, OR, USA
[c]Department of Radiation Medicine, Oregon Health and Science University, Portland, OR, USA

Lung cancer continues to be the leading cause of cancer-related mortality in both men and women [1]. Most lung cancers are diagnosed at an advanced stage, conferring a poor prognosis. Most patients who develop lung cancer smoke and have smoking-related damage to the heart and lungs, making the aggressive surgical or multimodality therapies involving surgery less viable options. Even in fit patients, survival outcomes with surgical resection alone in patients with locally advanced disease are poor [2]. The preponderance of patients with locally advanced non–small cell lung cancer (NSCLC) is treated with definitive chemoradiation without surgical resection. In fact about one third of newly diagnosed NSCLC patients have locally advanced disease that is not readily amenable to curative resection. The prognosis of these patients continues to be grim but with the improvement in staging techniques, improvement in radiation techniques, and the addition of newer chemotherapies, progress is being made.

Patients who present with locally advanced nonmetastatic NSCLC are a heterogeneous group that ranges from large tumors invading into the mediastinum with no lymph node involvement (T4 N0) to tumors with bulky multistation nodal involvement contralateral (N3) to the side of the primary neoplasm. A number of factors affect the outcome of these patients including involvement of lymph nodes, possible presence of undetected micrometastatic disease, lung function, weight loss, gender, and socioeconomic and performance status. This article covers pertinent issues related to systemic therapy and thoracic radiation therapy (TRT) in the definitive management of NSCLC.

Historical perspective

During the 1970s and 1980s, TRT alone was the standard of care for patients with medically inoperable or surgically unresectable locally advanced NSCLC. Based on the Radiation Therapy Oncology Group trial (RTOG) 73-01, a minimal tumor dose of 60 Gy in once-daily fractions of 2.0 Gy had been considered a standard dose for these patients. In this study, patients were randomized to receive 40, 50, or 60 Gy in a continuous fashion or 40 Gy in split-course fashion. The 2-year survival rate was 14% to 18% for patients treated continuously and only 10% for those treated in a split-course fashion. At 3 years, the survival rate was 15% to 20% for patients treated with 50 or 60 Gy versus 10% for patients in the 40-Gy group ($P = .10$). After 4 years, the survival was 4% to 6% in all groups. While local failure decreased as one increased dose, the rate of distant metastasis was greater than 75% in all groups [3]. We now can appreciate the strong likelihood that many patients likely harbored subclinical disease that was not readily detectable with the diagnostic armamentarium that was available in that practice era.

* Corresponding author.
E-mail address: Shilpenp@u.washington.edu (S. Patel).

doi:10.1016/j.thorsurg.2008.07.003

In an attempt to reduce distant failures, cytotoxic chemotherapy has been incorporated with radiation therapy. At least three meta-analyses showed a survival benefit when cisplatin-based (doublet or triplet) combination chemotherapy was combined with TRT [4–6]. Multiple trials have demonstrated an improvement in survival time with the addition of chemotherapy (commonly referred to as induction or neoadjuvant) given before TRT compared with TRT alone. Most notably, the Cancer and Leukemia Group B conducted a study (CALGB 8433) that compared standard TRT to 60 Gy with sequential cisplatin and vinblastine chemotherapy doublet for two cycles over 5 weeks followed by 60 Gy of TRT alone in patients with inoperable stage IIIA or IIIB disease. After 7 years of follow-up, the median survival time was 13.7 months versus 9.6 months ($P = .0066$) and the 7-year overall survival was 13% versus 6% favoring the addition of chemotherapy [7,8]. This trial was later confirmed by an Intergroup trial led by the RTOG (protocol 88-08), which compared TRT to 60 Gy, hyperfractionated TRT to 69.6 Gy, and sequential cisplatin and vinblastine doublet chemotherapy followed by 60 Gy of TRT [9]. The combined-modality arm once again demonstrated superiority when compared with either of the TRT-alone arms. Worth noting, the hyperfractionated arm was not superior to the conventional radiation therapy–alone arm. There are a number of trials that have demonstrated a benefit with the addition of chemotherapy; however, there have been trials where no benefit was seen [10]. Most of these trials are criticized because they use non–platinum-based chemotherapy and/or lacked the statistical power to demonstrate a significant advantage via a combined-modality approach.

With this information in hand, investigators began to try using chemotherapy concurrently (or concomitantly) with TRT. The European Organization for Research and Treatment of Cancer (EORTC) conducted a three-arm study that randomized patients to TRT alone to 55 Gy, TRT with weekly cisplatin, or TRT with low-dose daily cisplatin. The addition of concomitant chemotherapy to TRT improved 2-year survival from 13% to 19% in those patients who received weekly cisplatin and 26% in those patients who received daily cisplatin ($P = .009$) [11]. Although this study was positive, not all studies have returned to show a benefit. A study reported in 1992 led by Trovo and colleagues [12] randomized patients to a split-course of radiation therapy with and without the addition of daily cisplatin. Between January 1987 and June 1991, 173 patients with inoperable stage III NSCLC were entered into a randomized trial comparing TRT alone versus TRT and low-dose daily cisplatin (6 mg/m^2/day). An overall response rate of 59% was observed in patients who received TRT alone and 51% in patients who also received cisplatin. No differences in the pattern of relapse were noted between the two treatment groups. Median survivals were 10.3 months and 9.97 months, respectively. In this study, no significant advantage of the combined treatment over TRT only was found. The Hoosier Oncology Group confirmed this finding when they compared TRT alone with and without cisplatin every 3 weeks. In that study, Arm A consisted of TRT alone, 60 to 65 Gy total tumor dose, and arm B consisted of identical TRT with the addition of cisplatin 70 mg/m^2 every 3 weeks for three cycles beginning on the first day of irradiation. The median progression-free survival time was 23 versus 22 weeks, respectively ($P = .0537$). The median survival time was 43 weeks on the combination arm versus 46 weeks on the XRT arm (P overall = .3469). The 1-, 2-, and 5-year survival rates were 43%, 18%, and 5% on the combination arm versus 45%, 13%, and 2% on the XRT arm, respectively. The authors found that cisplatin, administered every 3 weeks, does not significantly improve response rate, progression-free survival, or overall survival when added to TRT for locally advanced unresectable NSCLC [13].

The next logical iteration of the combined-modality focus would be to compare concurrent versus sequential chemoradiation. The West Japan Lung Cancer Group compared patients receiving two cycles of induction (or neoadjuvant) mitomycin, vindesine, and cisplatin along with concomitant split-course TRT to a total dose of 56 Gy, to another cohort of individuals who received two cycles of the same chemotherapy followed by continuous course TRT to 56 Gy [14]. When chemotherapy was given with TRT concurrently, 5-year survival rates increased from 8.9% to 15.8%. ($P = .0001$). The authors attributed this improved survival to the increased local control [14]. The RTOG also completed a trial that compared hyperfractionated TRT to a total dose of 69.6 Gy with cisplatin and etoposide to standard TRT to 60 Gy with cisplatin and vinblastine given sequentially (similar to RTOG-8808 and CALGB-8433), and the same chemoradiation therapy concurrently. The median survival was 15.6 months in the hyperfractionated arm, 14.6 months in the sequential arm, to 17 months in the concurrent arm ($P = .046$). Acute toxicities of grade 3 or higher were 30% in the sequential arm, 48% in the concurrent chemotherapy with standard radiation therapy, and 62% in the concurrent chemotherapy and hyperfractionated radiation therapy. There was no statistically significant difference in late toxicities among the three arms [15]. Based on these trials and other studies, concurrent chemoradiation has become an accepted standard of care for patients with unresectable locally advanced NSCLC. Worth noting is that whereas survival is increased, toxicity is significantly higher in those patients who receive chemoradiation.

Induction versus consolidation chemotherapy

Given the survival advantages demonstrated with the sequential addition of systemic chemotherapy (induction) before definitive radiation, as well as the further improvement in survival with concurrent chemotherapy and radiation, a combination of the two approaches has been attractive to researchers. The combination of induction chemotherapy before concurrent definitive chemoradiation therapy has been investigated.

The CALGB investigated the addition of two cycles of cisplatin-based combination chemotherapy before the administration of two more cycles of the same doublet concurrent with definitive radiation (total dose 66 Gy) in patients with unresectable stage III NSCLC (CALGB 9431). In this randomized phase II study, 175 patients received cisplatin in combination with gemcitabine, paclitaxel, or vinorelbine. The median overall survival for all patients was 17 months (the study was not sufficiently powered to detect survival differences between the arms), and 3-year survival was 28%, 19%, and 23%, for gemcitabine, paclitaxel, and vinorelbine, respectively. The authors noted the results of this trial demonstrated an improvement over historical controls; however, historical controls had received sequential therapy. The authors concluded that further investigation of induction chemotherapy before concurrent definitive chemoradiation was warranted in a larger randomized trial [16].

In a nonrandomized phase II study of unresectable stage III NSCLC, Akerley and colleagues [17] evaluated two cycles of induction therapy with carboplatin and paclitaxel, followed by weekly low-dose carboplatin and paclitaxel concurrent with definitive radiotherapy to 66 Gy (CALGB 9534). The 3-year overall survival for the 40 eligible patients was 27%. Given the allowance for prior weight loss in this study, the authors concluded that the combination was feasible in an expanded trial population.

In one of the few phase III trials evaluating induction chemotherapy for locally advanced NSCLC, Kim and associates [18] randomized 134 patients with stage III NSCLC to receive two cycles of cisplatin and gemcitabine, followed by weekly cisplatin and paclitaxel concurrent with definitive radiotherapy, or definitive chemoradiotherapy alone. Median survival was 12.6 months with induction therapy, compared with 18.2 months on the control arm ($P = .18$), and progression-free survival was reported as 7.5 months versus 11.6 months in the control arm ($P = .04$). The authors concluded that induction chemotherapy failed to demonstrate a survival benefit compared with immediate chemoradiation, and instead demonstrated an inferior progression-free survival [18].

The CALGB conducted a randomized phase III trial comparing immediate concurrent chemoradiotherapy with weekly carboplatin and paclitaxel to two cycles of induction (neoadjuvant) chemotherapy with carboplatin and paclitaxel followed by the identical chemoradiotherapy in 366 patients with unresectable stage III NSCLC (CALGB 39801). Toxicities during concurrent therapy were similar, although patients undergoing induction therapy experienced toxicity related to the induction. No difference was detected in median survival between the two treatment arms (12 months versus 14 months, $P = .3$). The authors concluded that the addition of induction chemotherapy added toxicity without survival benefit over concurrent chemoradiotherapy alone. Additionally, given the poor median survival in this large study in both treatment arms, the investigators suggested that the use of weekly low-dose carboplatin and paclitaxel should be reexamined [19].

Other studies have investigated the addition of consolidation chemotherapy after the completion of definitive chemoradiotherapy. The Southwest Oncology Group conducted a phase II study of two cycles of cisplatin and etoposide administered with concurrent radiation for patients with surgically staged IIIB NSCLC (SWOG 9019). Patients subsequently were treated with two further cycles of consolidation cisplatin and etoposide. Median survival in the 50 eligible patients was 15 months, with a 15% 5-year survival reported initially. The authors concluded that given the feasibility and long-term survival, this combination was justified to be used as the control arm in future phase III studies [20].

The SWOG investigators subsequently evaluated the feasibility of altering the consolidation chemotherapy in an effort to overcome theoretic development of cross-resistance. Three cycles of docetaxel were substituted for the consolidation cisplatin and etoposide in a phase II study, SWOG 9504 (concurrent chemoradiation used the identical regimen as SWOG 9019). Median survival for the 83 eligible patients was 26 months, with 3-year survival reported initially as 37%. The authors concluded that the regimen was tolerable and the promising survival warranted evaluation in a phase III trial [21]. These conclusions were further supported by long-term follow-up of both studies, which noted 17% 5-year survival for patients in the SWOG 9019 study, and 29% 5-year survival for patients in the SWOG 9504 trial [22].

The SWOG 0023 trial was designed to be the phase III randomized trial to simultaneously confirm the results of the phase II study using cisplatin and etoposide with concurrent definitive radiation followed by three cycles of consolidation docetaxel, as well as to evaluate potential survival benefits of the addition of maintenance therapy with the epidermal growth factor receptor, gefitinib. Accrual was halted after an unplanned interim analysis of the 243 randomized patients (of 672 planned patients) demonstrated a rejection of the hypothesis of improved survival. Median survival for patients treated with maintenance gefitinib was 23 months, compared with 35 months for the control arm ($P =$ .013). The authors concluded that the addition of maintenance gefitinib after chemoradiation and consolidation docetaxel produced an inferior survival. As the rate of toxic death was not significantly increased and the most common cause of death was from lung cancer, the authors concluded that decreased survival was the result of tumor progression [23].

Belani and associates [24] conducted a three-arm randomized phase II trial in patients with locally advanced NSCLC (LAMP trial). The treatment arms consisted of two cycles of induction carboplatin and paclitaxel followed by definitive radiation (Arm 1); two cycles of the same induction chemotherapy followed by low-dose weekly carboplatin and paclitaxel administered concurrently with radiation (Arm 2); or concurrent chemoradiation followed by two cycles of consolidation carboplatin and paclitaxel (Arm 3). An interim analysis prompted closure of the second arm owing to the low likelihood of statistical benefit compared with historical controls. Accrual in the remaining treatment arms was subsequently expanded to accommodate a phase III design; however, with the emerging data of the superiority of concurrent therapy over sequential therapy, the trial was closed because of slowing accrual. For the 257 eligible patients, median survival was 13.0, 12.7, and 16.3 months, respectively, with no significant difference when compared with historical controls (RTOG 8808 sequential chemo- and radiotherapy study arm).

A randomized phase III study directly comparing the overall survival of cisplatin and etoposide with concurrent radiation with and without consolidation docetaxel for unresectable stage III NSCLC was performed by the Hoosier Oncology Group. The study was terminated owing to futility upon analysis of the initial 203 (of planned 259) patients enrolled. No differences were noted in progression-free survival between the treatment arms (12.3 months with consolidation versus 12.9 months control, $P = .941$), or in median survival (21.5 months with consolidation versus 24.1 months control, $P = .940$). Three-year survival was 27.2% and 27.6% for consolidation and controls, respectively ($P =$ nonsignificant). Rates of hospitalization, infection, and treatment-related death were significantly higher in the consolidation arm, leading the investigators to conclude that consolidation chemotherapy does not contribute to survival benefit, but does incur increased toxicity compared with chemoradiotherapy [25].

The studies evaluating induction and consolidation chemotherapy administered around definitive chemoradiation have, for the most part, been smaller phase II trials. Unfortunately at this time, the evidence in both phase II and phase III studies indicates that neither approach improves survival over concurrent chemoradiation alone. Indeed, in the case of gefitinib, the addition of maintenance therapy decreases survival [23]. The mechanisms for inferior survival with gefitinib maintenance therapy are not understood. Given the current data, the addition of either induction or consolidation chemotherapy is not recommended outside of the clinical trial setting.

Chemotherapy options: carboplatin versus cisplatin

The optimal chemotherapeutic regimen to use with concurrent radiation has not been definitively established. Platinum-based combinations are the most commonly used, although debate exists between the use of carboplatin and cisplatin. There has never been a randomized trial comparing cisplatin- and carboplatin-based regimens with definitive TRT powered for detection of survival outcomes. This makes inferences of relative superiority of survivals between existing studies difficult. Given the more favorable toxicity profile of carboplatin, weekly carboplatin and paclitaxel is one of the most popular regimens used in the United States, although the results of CALGB 39801 call this practice into question [19]. The long-term outcomes of the SWOG cisplatin-based regimens demonstrate some of the most consistent survival rates, with median survivals ranging from 24 to 35 months [21,23,25]. Thus, the combination of cisplatin and etoposide is recognized as the standard of care for future chemoradiation studies for both SWOG and ECOG.

Treatment options for special populations

Most clinical trials for NSCLC require patients to have a good baseline performance status (Zubrod 0–1) before enrollment, including the chemoradiation studies discussed earlier in this article. A recent analysis indicates that between 34% and 48% of patients with lung cancer have a poor performance status [26]. The exclusion of patients with poor performance status (Zubrod status 2–4) leads to a lack of evidence with which to treat a significant portion of patients with NSCLC.

SWOG has conducted phase II studies evaluating definitive chemoradiation in poor-risk patients. In the SWOG trial 9429, 60 poor-risk patients with stage III NSCLC were treated with definitive concurrent carboplatin, etoposide, and TRT. "Poor-risk" disease criteria included chronic obstructive pulmonary disease (COPD) with poor pulmonary function (72% of enrolled patients), limited renal function with creatinine clearance less than 50 mL/min (12%), hearing loss (13%), peripheral neuropathy (8%), controlled congestive heart failure at risk for decompensation (12%), tumor-induced weight loss, low albumin, or performance status of 2 (17% of the latter three combined). No treatment-related deaths were seen. Median overall survival was 13 months, and 2-year survival was 21%. The investigators concluded that the regimen was well tolerated in poor-risk patients otherwise ineligible for enrollment into standard-risk clinical trials, and that further studies were warranted [27].

The SWOG 9712 study subsequently examined the addition of three cycles of consolidation paclitaxel after completion of the regimen described in the preceding paragraph in a phase II study using the same entry criteria. In the 87 patients eligible for evaluation, 38% had performance status 2, weight loss, or low albumin. Poor pulmonary function accounted for 31%, impaired renal function for 13%, hearing loss for 15%, and congestive heart failure for 3% of the enrolled patients. Contrary to the results of the previous study, this trial demonstrated an unacceptable rate of toxicity including toxic death, with three patients (3% of total population) suffering grade 5 complications during chemoradiation and an additional four patients (7.5% of patients evaluable) suffering grade 5 complications during consolidation therapy. Overall survival was not improved (10.2 months), and 2-year survival was 25%. The authors concluded that the addition of consolidation paclitaxel significantly increased toxicity without improving survival, and that more stringent eligibility criteria would need to be applied during future trials involving patients with poor-risk NSCLC [28].

Currently, no consensus standard therapy exists for patients with poor-risk locally advanced NSCLC. Patients with poor performance status; impaired pulmonary, cardiac, or renal function; baseline neuropathy; or hearing loss, or other comorbid illnesses may be candidates for curative therapy, although the risk of toxicity is clearly increased. Given the paucity of data, a tailored approach may be required at this time, including the use of renal-sparing agents such as carboplatin. An ongoing feasibility study (SWOG 0429) is evaluating the combination of low-dose docetaxel and the monoclonal antibody to the epidermal growth factor receptor, cetuximab, in combination with definitive radiation for patients with poor-risk disease [29]. It is hoped that the newer molecularly targeted agents may offer therapeutic benefit with a relatively lower toxicity profile.

Radiation planning and delivery

One of the challenges of treating patients with lung cancer is the ability to accurately target the tumor. Previous efforts to use two-dimensional tumor planning have resulted in a less than ideal outcome. Fortunately, multiple technological advances have occurred recently that will hopefully allow radiation oncologists to more accurately target the tumor and increase the ability to improve local control, while enhancing the overall therapeutic ratio. Ideally one would like to increase the probability of local control but be mindful of the fact that as one increases dose the probability of complications also increases (Fig. 1). The advent of three-dimensional treatment planning allows one to delineate the target and avoid the normal structures in the lung. In addition to planning, most modern treatment planning systems allow for the fusion of anatomic datasets (ie, computed tomography [CT], magnetic resonance imaging [MRI]) with functional imaging datasets such as 18-fluorodeoxyglucose (FDG) positron emission tomography (PET), which helps delineate a more biologically relevant tumor target, as opposed to noncancerous tissue such as postobstruction atelectasis. This modality can also be used midtreatment to aid in treatment adjustments for target volume shift during a course of TRT, referred to as adaptive radiotherapy. One must be careful with this new technology though, as the use of PET scans in treatment planning purposes continues to be evaluated and validated in terms of its accuracy of depicting true tumor extent. Also, many centers are now able to simulate patients in a four-dimensional CT unit. This allows oncologists to track the tumor in all directions over time. Patients are usually evaluated retrospectively over each of the breathing cycles. This evaluation allows the clinician to make adjustments as a result of respiratory motion for treatment planning purposes. Major improvements in radiation treatment planning continue to evolve and allow oncologists to better delineate tumors and accurately treat patients.

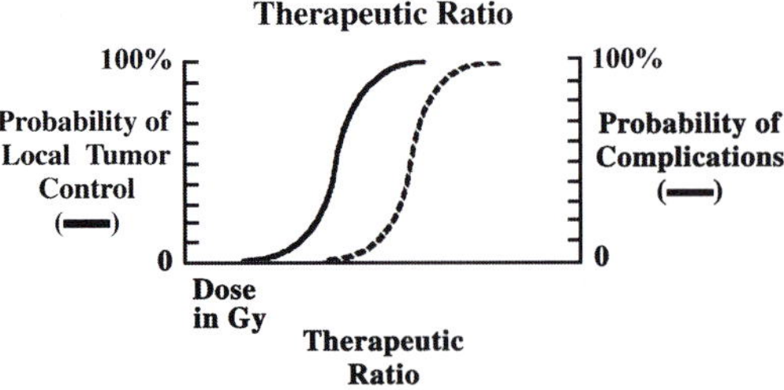

Fig. 1. The relationship between the two curves represents the therapeutic ratio. As one increases the probability of tumor control, the probability of complications also increases.

Tumor dose

One of the basic principles in radiation oncology historically is that doses in the range of 80 to 100 Gy are required to sterilize tumors [30]. Given the fragile nature of lung tissue and other tissues in the surrounding area, this is difficult to achieve in NSCLC. With improved radiation planning in lung cancer, efforts have been made to determine if dose escalation delivered with chemotherapy can improve outcomes. One of the first studies reported was from the University of North Carolina–based consortium, in which investigators conducted a phase I/II study that escalated the dose of TRT from 60 Gy to 74 Gy. All patients received a cycle of induction chemotherapy before going on to concurrent chemoradiation. The chemotherapy regimen both in the induction and concurrent arms was carboplatin and paclitaxel. The median survival time was 24 months [31]. The RTOG (protocol 93-11) followed suit and conducted a trial with weekly paclitaxel and carboplatin and concurrent dose escalated thoracic radiation therapy. The Phase I study began at a dose level of 75.25 Gy in 2.15-Gy once-daily fractions prescribed to the isocenter. Three patients in the first cohort developed dose-limiting pulmonary toxicity. The dose was then deescalated to 74 Gy in 2-Gy daily fractions. The median survival time for the patients who received 74 Gy was 22 months [32]. The North Central Cancer Treatment Group had also reported the results of a phase I radiation dose escalation trial. All patients received weekly paclitaxel and carboplatin with an initial radiation dose of 70 Gy in daily 2-Gy fractions. The maximum tolerated dose was determined to be 74 Gy. In this study, the median survival time was 37 months [33]. Because of these and other studies [34], the RTOG has proposed a study evaluating conformal radiation therapy to 60 Gy compared with 74 Gy with chemotherapy.

Future directions

The treatment of locally advanced NSCLC is complex, and although significant gains have been made in survival in the past few decades, outcomes are still poor and long-term survival is low. Ongoing studies are crucial if further improvement is to be made. The many potential avenues of ongoing investigation include optimization of radiation dose and delivery, application of newer chemotherapeutic agents in combination with definitive radiation, and the use of molecularly targeted agents.

The CALGB 30105 study has evaluated high-dose three-dimensional conformal radiation to 74 Gy in combination with chemotherapy. In this randomized phase II study, 69 patients received two cycles of induction chemotherapy with either carboplatin and paclitaxel or carboplatin with gemcitabine, followed by concurrent radiation with the same regimen. The gemcitabine-containing treatment arm was closed prematurely because of a high rate of grade 5 toxicity (three grade 5 pulmonary events, 13%). Median progression-free survival has been reported as 15.2 months. Further maturation of the data is awaited for reporting of median survival [35].

An ongoing phase III trial is directly comparing high-dose conformal thoracic radiation (74 Gy) versus standard radiation (60 Gy) for patients with unresectable stage III NSCLC. Patients will receive concurrent carboplatin and paclitaxel, followed by consolidation carboplatin and paclitaxel after the completion of chemoradiation (RTOG 0617) [29].

Newer chemotherapeutic agents, such as pemetrexed, are currently undergoing evaluation in combination with cisplatin and definitive radiation for unresectable stage III NSCLC [29]. It is hoped that the lower toxicity profile in relation to other systemic chemotherapeutic agents may improve tolerability, and perhaps outcomes, for patients with locally advanced disease [36].

Despite the adverse outcome of the SWOG 0023 study [23], investigation with agents targeted against the epidermal growth factor receptor (EGFR) are ongoing in the setting of locally advanced disease. Cetuximab is undergoing evaluation in combination with radiation after platinum-based induction chemotherapy for patients with stage III NSCLC (the SCRATCH study) [37]. A randomized phase III trial of maintenance therapy with the EGFR tyrosine kinase inhibitor erlotinib after definitive chemoradiation (using carboplatin and docetaxel) is ongoing [29].

Efforts to identify those patients with NSCLC most likely to benefit from therapy, and those most likely to have resistant disease, have shown progress in the past few years through a variety of molecular analytic approaches. In patients with advanced NSCLC, elevated tumor expression of ERCC1, a DNA repair enzyme, is associated with cisplatin resistance [38]. In resected early-stage disease, patients with elevated ERCC1 expression do not experience a survival benefit with adjuvant cisplatin-based chemotherapy [39]. Tumors with elevated expression of RRM1, the molecular target of gemcitabine chemotherapy, have been shown to have an inverse response to gemcitabine therapy [40]. ERCC1 and RRM1 are reviewed in further detail in the article on adjuvant therapy for N2 disease in this journal. Ongoing prospective evaluations in advanced NSCLC tailoring chemotherapy regimens based on ERCC1 and RRM1 expression are ongoing [41]. If a survival advantage with tailoring chemotherapy is shown, further evaluation with definitive chemotherapy will be warranted.

Multiple other molecular evaluations are under investigation. In an analysis of the adjuvant chemotherapy trial JBR.10, a 15-gene expression profile was identified that separated 62 patients in the observation group into high-risk and low-risk groups for death ($P < .0001$). In validation sets, chemotherapy was shown to reduce the risk of death after surgical resection for high-risk patients, regardless of tumor stage [42]. Other investigators have identified a five-gene expression signature predictive for outcome in early-stage resected NSCLC adjusted for tumor histology, and a three-gene expression signature predictive for survival outcome without adjustment for histology [43]. A tumor amplicon set with gene expression of TTF-1, NKX2-8, and PAX9, that has prognostic value for survival and predictive value for cisplatin resistance, has been identified [44]. These predictive and prognostic studies need further evaluation in large prospective trials before clinical application. Questions regarding which profile, or combination of profiles, will be optimal still need to be addressed. If an optimal profile is identified for use in the adjuvant setting, this may then be further investigated in application toward tailoring therapy in locally advanced disease.

Summary

The treatment of NSCLC continues to evolve over time. Newer therapies and techniques help achieve success in this difficult disease. Since the 1970s, one can observe trends in median survival and notice that they have improved from 9 to 10 months to now 15 to 24 months with concurrent chemoradiation. Unfortunately, despite the advances made, most patients still die from their disease. Chemoradiation without induction or consolidation therapy continues to remain the standard of care in this country for unresectable locally advanced NSCLC. Evaluation of epidermal growth factor receptor tyrosine kinase inhibitors and other biologics continue to be investigated but are not considered standard of care yet. Technologies continue to expand including the use of four-dimensional CT scans and PET scans to more accurately plan patients. Future application of molecular profiling to predict patients most likely to benefit from tailored chemotherapeutic approaches is awaited following validation in early- and advanced-stage disease. With continued diligence to testing new ideas in NSCLC, it is hoped that outcomes will continue to improve the lives of patients with this devastating disease.

References

[1] Jemal A, Siegel R, Ward E, et al. Cancer statistics, 2007. CA Cancer J Clin 2007;57:43–66.

[2] Roth JA, Atkinson EN, Fossella F, et al. Long-term follow-up of patients enrolled in a randomized trial comparing perioperative chemotherapy and surgery with surgery alone in resectable stage IIIA non-small-cell lung cancer. Lung Cancer 1998;21:1–6.

[3] Perez CA, Pajak TF, Rubin P, et al. Long-term observations of the patterns of failure in patients with unresectable non-oat cell carcinoma of the lung treated with definitive radiotherapy. Report by the Radiation Therapy Oncology Group. Cancer 1987;59:1874–81.

[4] Chemotherapy in non-small cell lung cancer: a meta-analysis using updated data on individual patients from 52 randomised clinical trials. Non-small Cell Lung Cancer Collaborative Group. BMJ 1995;311:899–909.

[5] Pritchard RS, Anthony SP. Chemotherapy plus radiotherapy compared with radiotherapy alone in the treatment of locally advanced, unresectable, non-small-cell lung cancer. A meta-analysis. Ann Intern Med 1996;125:723–9.

[6] Marino P, Preatoni A, Cantoni A. Randomized trials of radiotherapy alone versus combined chemotherapy and radiotherapy in stages IIIa and IIIb nonsmall cell lung cancer. A meta-analysis. Cancer 1995;76:593–601.

[7] Dillman RO, Herndon J, Seagren SL, et al. Improved survival in stage III non-small-cell lung cancer: seven-year follow-up of Cancer and Leukemia Group B (CALGB) 8433 trial. J Natl Cancer Inst 1996;88:1210–5.

[8] Dillman RO, Seagren SL, Propert KJ, et al. A randomized trial of induction chemotherapy plus high-dose radiation versus radiation alone in stage III non-small-cell lung cancer. N Engl J Med 1990;323:940–5.

[9] Sause W, Kolesar P, Taylor SI, et al. Final results of phase III trial in regionally advanced unresectable non-small cell lung cancer: Radiation Therapy Oncology Group, Eastern Cooperative Oncology Group, and Southwest Oncology Group. Chest 2000;117:358–64.

[10] Morton RF, Jett JR, McGinnis WL, et al. Thoracic radiation therapy alone compared with combined chemoradiotherapy for locally unresectable non-small cell lung cancer. A randomized, phase III trial. Ann Intern Med 1991;115:681–6.

[11] Schaake-Koning C, van den Bogaert W, Dalesio O, et al. Effects of concomitant cisplatin and radiotherapy on inoperable non-small-cell lung cancer. N Engl J Med 1992;326:524–30.

[12] Trovo MG, Zanelli GD, Minatel E, et al. Radiotherapy versus radiotherapy enhanced by cisplatin in stage III non-small cell lung cancer. Int J Radiat Oncol Biol Phys 1992;24:573–4.

[13] Blanke C, Ansari R, Mantravadi R, et al. Phase III trial of thoracic irradiation with or without cisplatin for locally advanced unresectable non-small-cell lung cancer: a Hoosier Oncology Group protocol. J Clin Oncol 1995;13:1425–9.

[14] Furuse K, Fukuoka M, Kawahara M, et al. Phase III study of concurrent versus sequential thoracic radiotherapy in combination with mitomycin, vindesine, and cisplatin in unresectable stage III non-small-cell lung cancer. J Clin Oncol 1999;17:2692–9.

[15] Curran WJ, SC, Langer C, et al. Phase III comparison of sequential versus concurrent chemoradiation for patients with unresected stage III non small cell lung cancer: initial report of RTOG 9410. Proceedings of the American Society of Clinical Oncology 2000;19:484a.

[16] Vokes EE, Herndon JE 2nd, Crawford J, et al. Randomized phase II study of cisplatin with gemcitabine or paclitaxel or vinorelbine as induction chemotherapy followed by concomitant chemoradiotherapy for stage IIIB non-small-cell lung cancer: cancer and leukemia group B study 9431. J Clin Oncol 2002;20:4191–8.

[17] Akerley W, Herndon JE Jr, Lyss AP, et al. Induction paclitaxel/carboplatin followed by concurrent chemoradiation therapy for unresectable stage III non-small-cell lung cancer: a limited-access study–CALGB 9534. Clin Lung Cancer 2005;7:47–53.

[18] Kim S, KM, Choi E, et al. Induction chemotherapy followed by concurrent chemoradiotherapy (CCRT) versus CCRT alone for unresectable stage III non-small cell lung cancer: randomized phase III trial. Proc Am Soc Clin Oncol 2007;25:7528.

[19] Vokes EE, Herndon JE 2nd, Kelley MJ, et al. Induction chemotherapy followed by chemoradiotherapy compared with chemoradiotherapy alone for regionally advanced unresectable stage III non-small-cell lung cancer: Cancer and Leukemia Group B. J Clin Oncol 2007;25:1698–704.

[20] Albain KS, Crowley JJ, Turrisi AT 3rd, et al. Concurrent cisplatin, etoposide, and chest radiotherapy

in pathologic stage IIIB non-small-cell lung cancer: a Southwest Oncology Group phase II study, SWOG 9019. J Clin Oncol 2002;20:3454–60.
[21] Gandara DR, Chansky K, Albain KS, et al. Consolidation docetaxel after concurrent chemoradiotherapy in stage IIIB non-small-cell lung cancer: phase II Southwest Oncology Group Study S9504. J Clin Oncol 2003;21:2004–10.
[22] Gandara DR, CK, Albain KS, et al. Long-term survival with concurrent chemoradiation therapy followed by consolidation docetaxel in stage IIIB non-small-cell lung cancer: a phase II Southwest Oncology Group study (S9504). Clin Lung Cancer 2006;8:116–21.
[23] Kelly K, Chansky K, Gaspar LE, et al. Phase III trial of maintenance gefitinib or placebo after concurrent chemoradiotherapy and docetaxel consolidation in inoperable stage III non-small-cell lung cancer: SWOG S0023. J Clin Oncol 2008;26(15):2450–6.
[24] Belani CP, Choy H, Bonomi P, et al. Combined chemoradiotherapy regimens of paclitaxel and carboplatin for locally advanced non-small-cell lung cancer: a randomized phase II locally advanced multi-modality protocol. J Clin Oncol 2005;23: 5883–91.
[25] Hanna NH, NM, Ansari R, et al. Phase III trial of cisplatin plus etoposide plus concurrent chest radiation with or without consolidation docetaxel in patients with inoperable stage III non-small cell lung cancer: HOG LUN 01-24/USO-023. Proc Am Soc Clin Oncol 2007;25:7512.
[26] Lilenbaum RC, Cashy J, Hensing TA, et al. Prevalence of poor performance status in lung cancer patients: implications for research. J Thorac Oncol 2008;3:125–9.
[27] Lau DH, Crowley JJ, Gandara DR, et al. Southwest Oncology Group phase II trial of concurrent carboplatin, etoposide, and radiation for poor-risk stage III non-small-cell lung cancer. J Clin Oncol 1998; 16:3078–81.
[28] Davies AM, Chansky K, Lau DH, et al. Phase II study of consolidation paclitaxel after concurrent chemoradiation in poor-risk stage III non-small-cell lung cancer: SWOG S9712. J Clin Oncol 2006; 24:5242–6.
[29] National Cancer Institute. Available at: www.cancer.gov. Accessed September 2008.
[30] Fletcher GH. Clinical dose response curves of human malignant epithelial tumours. Br J Radiol 1973;46:151.
[31] Socinski MA, Rosenman JG, Halle J, et al. Dose-escalating conformal thoracic radiation therapy with induction and concurrent carboplatin/paclitaxel in unresectable stage IIIA/B nonsmall cell lung carcinoma: a modified phase I/II trial. Cancer 2001;92: 1213–23.
[32] Bradley J, Graham MV, Winter K, et al. Toxicity and outcome results of RTOG 9311: a phase I-II dose-escalation study using three-dimensional conformal radiotherapy in patients with inoperable non-small-cell lung carcinoma. Int J Radiat Oncol Biol Phys 2005;61:318–28.
[33] Schild SE, Wong WW, Vora SA, et al. The long-term results of a pilot study of three times a day radiotherapy and escalating doses of daily cisplatin for locally advanced non-small-cell lung cancer. Int J Radiat Oncol Biol Phys 2005;62:1432–7.
[34] Blackstock AW, Ho C, Butler J, et al. Phase Ia/Ib chemo-radiation trial of gemcitabine and dose-escalated thoracic radiation in patients with stage III A/B non-small cell lung cancer. J Thorac Oncol 2006;1: 434–40.
[35] Blackstock AW, SM, Bogart J, et al. Induction plus concurrent chemotherapy with high-dose (74 Gy) 3-dimensional thoracic radiotherapy in stage III non-small cell lung cancer: preliminary report of Cancer and Leukemia Group B (CALGB) 30105. Proc Am Soc Clin Oncol 2006;24:7042.
[36] Hanna N, Shepherd FA, Fossella FV, et al. Randomized phase III trial of pemetrexed versus docetaxel in patients with non-small-cell lung cancer previously treated with chemotherapy. J Clin Oncol 2004;22:1589–97.
[37] Hughes SR, LJ, Miah A, et al. Safety study of induction chemotherapy and synchronous radiotherapy and cetuximab in stage III non-small cell lung cancer: SCRATCH (Cohort 1). Proc Am Soc Clin Oncol 2007;25:18032.
[38] Lord RV, Brabender J, Gandara D, et al. Low ERCC1 expression correlates with prolonged survival after cisplatin plus gemcitabine chemotherapy in non-small cell lung cancer. Clin Cancer Res 2002;8:2286–91.
[39] Olaussen KA, Dunant A, Fouret P, et al. DNA repair by ERCC1 in non-small-cell lung cancer and cisplatin-based adjuvant chemotherapy. N Engl J Med 2006;355:983–91.
[40] Bepler G, Kusmartseva I, Sharma S, et al. RRM1 modulated in vitro and in vivo efficacy of gemcitabine and platinum in non-small-cell lung cancer. J Clin Oncol 2006;24:4731–7.
[41] Simon GR, WC, Chiappori AA, et al. Molecular analysis-directed individualized therapy (MADeIT) in advanced non-small cell lung cancer. Proc Am Soc Clin Oncol 2007;25:7502.
[42] Tsao MS, ZC, Ding K, et al. A 15-gene expression signature prognostic for survival and predictive for adjuvant chemotherapy benefit in JBR.10 patients. Proc Am Soc Clin Oncol 2008;26:7510.
[43] Skrzypski M, JE, Benlloch S, et al. Validation of 5- and 3-gene expression signatures for predicting outcome in non-small cell lung cancer patients. Proc Am Soc Clin Oncol 2008;26:7532.
[44] Hsu SD, AC, Riedel RF, et al. Use of co-activation of lung cancer specific developmental pathway genes, TTF-1, NKX2-8, and PAX9, to predict prognosis and guide therapeutic strategies. Proc Am Soc Clin Oncol 2008;26:7511.

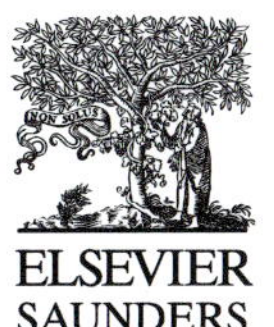

ELSEVIER
SAUNDERS

Thorac Surg Clin 18 (2008) 403–415

THORACIC
SURGERY
CLINICS

Neoadjuvant Therapy for Resectable Non–Small Cell Lung Cancer with Mediastinal Lymph Node Involvement

Brandon H. Tieu, MD[a], Rachel E. Sanborn, MD[b,*], Charles R. Thomas, Jr., MD[c]

[a]*Department of Surgery, Oregon Health and Science University, 3181 S.W. Sam Jackson Park Road, Portland, OR 97239, USA*

[b]*Department of Medical Oncology, Providence Portland Medical Center, 4805 N.E. Glisan Street, 2N35, Portland, OR 97213, USA*

[c]*Department of Radiation Medicine, Oregon Health and Science University, 3181 S.W. Sam Jackson Park Road, Portland, OR 97239, USA*

It is estimated that more than 215,000 men and women will be diagnosed with, and almost 162,000 men and women will die of, lung cancer in 2008 [1]. Between 10% and 37% of patients with non–small cell lung cancer (NSCLC) will present with ipsilateral mediastinal lymph node metastases (N2 disease) [2,3]. Both prognosis and treatment strategy are based on the extension of the disease to the mediastinum.

Historically, primary surgical therapy for stage IIIA NSCLC had poor 5-year survival rates, ranging betweeen 7% and 16% [4]. Adjuvant chemotherapy has been complicated by poor tolerance and decreased ability to complete therapy in the setting of surgical therapy.

Neoadjuvant therapy offers several potential benefits. Patients may be able to tolerate the chemotherapy regimen better because they are not recovering from surgery. Increased compliance and completion of planned therapy may result in decreased tumor burden and eradication of mediastinal disease allowing for complete resection. Distant micrometastatic disease can be treated early. Potential disadvantages include the development of medical illness and treatment-related toxicity. This may delay surgery or eliminate eligibility as a surgical candidate. In-addition, the accuracy of surgical staging may be affected by the treatment.

Mediastinal staging

The prognosis and optimal treatment of patients diagnosed with NSCLC depends on accurate staging [2,5–7]. Nodal involvement can be determined by either noninvasive or invasive measures. Although on computerized tomography (CT) imaging a lymph node larger than 1 cm in diameter is considered abnormal, studies have shown that size is not a reliable predictor of tumor involvement [8,9]. Toloza and colleagues [10] reported in a meta-analysis of 3438 patients imaged with CT a sensitivity of 0.57 (95% confidence interval [CI], 0.49–0.66), specificity of 0.82 (95% CI, 0.77–0.86), positive predictive value (PPV) 0.56 (range, 0.26 to 0.84), and negative predictive value (NPV) 0.83 (range, 0.63 to 0.93). Staging of the mediastinum by positron emission tomography (PET) in 1045 patients in the same meta-analysis had a pooled sensitivity of 0.84 (95% CI, 0.78–0.89), specificity of 0.89 (95% CI, 0.83–0.93), PPV of 0.79 (range, 0.4 to 1.00), NPV of 0.93 (range, 0.75 to 1.00). A meta-analysis by Birim and associates [11] compared CT and fluorodeoxyglucose (FDG)-PET for nodal staging and found an overall sensitivity and specificity of

* Corresponding author.
E-mail address: rachel.sanborn@providence.org (R.E. Sanborn).

doi:10.1016/j.thorsurg.2008.07.004

83% and 92%, respectively, for FDG-PET compared with an overall sensitivity and specificity of 59% and 78%, respectively, for CT scans. Fusion of CT and PET has been shown to increase accuracy over either modality used separately or in combination, and this technique may be used in patients with potentially resectable tumors to help direct nodal sampling [12].

Invasive nodal sampling can be performed by transbronchial (bronchoscopic or endobronchial ultrasound) needle aspiration (TBNA), transthoracic needle aspiration (TTNA), endoscopic ultrasound needle aspiration (EUS-NA), or mediastinoscopy. Toloza and colleagues [13] reported the sensitivity, specificity, and accuracy of negative lymph node biopsies of these methods from a pooled meta-analysis of 7015 patients. TTNA had the highest sensitivity 0.91 (95% CI, 0.74–0.91) followed by EUS-NA, medistinoscopy, and TBNA with sensitivities of 0.88 (95% CI, 0.82–0.93), 0.81 (95% CI, 0.76–0.85), and 0.76 (95% CI, 0.72–0.79), respectively. Mediastinoscopy had the highest NPV of 0.91 (range, 58%–97%) followed by TTNA, EUS-NA, and TBNA with NPVs of 0.78, 0.77, and 0.71, respectively. Although invasive clinical staging of the mediastinum can be effectively performed by any of these methods with similar sensitivities, there may be a selection bias. TTNA and EUS-NA are usually performed in patients with radiographic evidence that mediastinal lymphadenopathy is accessible by a biopsy needle. The NPVs are quite different, thus providing greater confidence in a negative lymph node biopsy on mediastinoscopy.

Induction chemotherapy

Numerous nonrandomized phase II trials using induction chemotherapy can be found in the literature. In a summary by Meko and Rusch [14], chemotherapy followed by surgery in highly selected patients with and without postoperative radiation therapy suggested there may be an improvement in resectability and possibly improved survival over single-modality therapy. Martini and colleagues [15] published their experience with the administration of two to three cycles of cisplatin, vindesine or vinblastine, and mitomycin followed by surgical resection. Patients with positive mediastinal nodes at thoracotomy received postoperative radiation, while all patients received two further cycles of adjuvant chemotherapy. Of the 136 patients in the study, 105 (77%) of 136 had a major response to induction therapy and complete resection was achieved in 89 (65%) of 136 patients. The median survival was 19 months and overall 3-year survival was 28%, representing an improvement over historical controls (8% 3-year survival).

Phase III studies evaluating neoadjuvant chemotherapy and surgery versus surgery alone date back to early 1990s. Neoadjuvant phase III trial results are summarized in Table 1.

Rosell and associates [16] randomized 60 patients with resectable NSCLC to receive surgery alone or three cycles of mitomycin, ifosfamide, and cisplatin followed by surgery. All patients received mediastinal radiation following surgery. Forty-four patients enrolled had N2 disease, although many patients were clinically staged only before surgery. Trial enrollment was prematurely halted after 24 months, when an interim analysis demonstrated significant survival differences between the two arms. Median survival was 26 months for the chemotherapy plus surgery arm compared with 8 months for surgery alone ($P < .001$). A significant difference in disease-free survival between the groups (20 months versus 5 months, $P < .001$) was also seen. In a subsequent long-term follow up analysis [17], overall median survival was 22 months for patients receiving neoadjuvant chemotherapy (versus 10 months with surgery alone, $P = .005$). Five-year survival was 17% with neoadjuvant chemotherapy, compared with 0% with surgery alone (P value not reported).

Roth and the group from MD Anderson Cancer Center [18] performed a similar study randomizing 60 patients to receive surgery alone or three cycles of chemotherapy with cyclosphosphamide, etoposide, and cisplatin followed by surgery. Patients with tumor regression received three more cycles of adjuvant chemotherapy. Postoperative radiotherapy was an option for patients with incomplete resections. In the neoadjuvant chemotherapy arm, 53% received adjuvant radiation, and 59% of patients in the surgery-alone arm received adjuvant radiation. Eighty-five percent of the patients were invasively staged (mediastinoscopy or mediastinotomy) before treatment. Trial enrollment was halted after 60 of the planned 130 patients were accrued given the results of an interim analysis indicating a significant survival benefit with induction therapy. The estimated median survival was 64 months compared with 11 months for the induction group and surgery-only group, respectively ($P = .018$).

Table 1
Phase III induction chemotherapy trials

Primary author	Disease stage	No. of patients	Regimen	Median survival	*P* value
Rosell [16,17]	Resectable	60	MIP × 3 → S vs S alone Adjuvant RT	CT→ S: 22mo S: 10 mo 5-y Surv: CT→S 17% S: 0%	.005
Roth [18]	IIIA	60	Cyclophos/EP × 3 → S → (Cyclophos/EP × 3 for responders) vs S alone	Est: CT→S→CT: 64 mo S: 11 mo Est 3-y Surv: CT→S →CT: 56% S: 15%	.018 NR
Pass [19]	IIIA (N2 disease)	27	EP × 2→S→ EP × 4 vs S→RT	CT→S→CT: 28.7 mo S→RT: 15.6 mo	.095
DePierre [20]	IB-IIIA	355	MIP × 2→S→MIP × 2 vs S alone	CT→S→CT: 37 mo S: 26 mo 4-y Surv: CT→S→CT: 44% S: 35%	.15 NR

Abbreviations: CT, chemotherapy; Cyclophos, cyclophosphamide; E, etoposide; Est, estimated; I, ifosfamide; M, mitomycin; Mo, months; NR, not reported; P, cisplatin; RT, radiation; S, surgery; 5-y Surv, 5-year survival.

In addition, the estimated 3-year survival rate favored the induction group (56% versus 15%, *P* value not reported). Interpretation of these studies has been difficult owing to the small sample sizes, inclusion of T3N0 and T3N1 tumors, variability of invasive staging, and the application of postoperative radiation therapy.

Not all neoadjuvant chemotherapy trials have shown a benefit compared with primary surgery. Pass and associates [19] randomized 27 patients with biopsy-proven N2 lymph node involvement to receive either two cycles of preoperative cisplatin and etoposide and then surgical resection followed by four more cycles of cisplatin and etoposide; or surgery followed by radiation therapy. The study was terminated early owing to poor accrual. An interim analysis however showed a trend toward increased survival in the induction chemotherapy group compared with the surgery and radiation group (median survival 28.7 months versus 15.6 months, $P = .095$).

Depierre and the French Thoracic Cooperative Group [20] conducted the largest study of neoadjuvant therapy in resectable NSCLC. The investigators randomized 355 clinically staged patients with stage I (except for T1N0), II, or IIIA histologically proven NSCLC (122 patients had N2 disease, including bulky disease) to induction chemotherapy consisting of two cycles of mitomycin, ifosfamide, and cisplatin followed by surgery, and two more cycles of the same chemotherapy; or to primary surgery alone. Patients with pT3 or pN2 disease as well as those with incomplete resections received adjuvant radiotherapy. A high number of pneumonectomies were performed in each group (55.7% in the primary surgery group and 48.6% in the preoperative chemotherapy plus surgery group). The overall median survival was 37 months for the chemotherapy group and 26 months in the primary surgery group ($P = .15$). In a subset analysis of patients with baseline N0 or N1 disease, survival favored the chemotherapy arm (hazard ratio 0.68, $P = .027$) over surgery alone. The same analysis did not show a survival benefit in the neoadjuvant chemotherapy group for patients with N2 disease (RR 1.04, $P = .85$).

Conclusive evidence regarding neoadjuvant chemotherapy for patients with N2 disease with the use of older chemotherapeutic regimens is thus lacking. The small number of patients enrolled in the positive phase III studies diminish broader applicability, however they do justify the ongoing investigation of more modern chemotherapeutic combinations in the neoadjuvant setting.

Induction chemotherapy with third-generation agents

Phase II trials evaluating the efficacy of third-generation chemotherapy agents have been performed with varying results. Results of studies evaluating induction chemotherapy with third-generation agents are summarized in Table 2.

The Swiss Group for Clinical Cancer Research (SAKK) enrolled 90 patients in a nonrandomized trial to receive three cycles of cisplatin and docetaxel followed by surgery. Postoperative radiation was given to 33 patients with positive surgical margins, with involvement of the highest mediastinal nodes, as well as at investigator discretion. The investigators reported an overall response rate of 66%, with a 19% complete pathological response rate in the 78 patients undergoing surgical resection. Forty-eight percent of the 87 patients assessable by intention-to-treat analysis underwent a complete resection. Median survival was 27.6 months. The 3-year survival for patients downstaged to N0 or N1 status with induction chemotherapy was 61%, whereas 3-year survival for those patients with persistent N2 disease at the time of surgery was only 11%. The authors concluded that patients without mediastinal downstaging at the time of surgery did not benefit from surgical resection [21].

De Marinis and colleagues [22] treated 49 patients with three cycles of cisplatin, gemcitabine, and paclitaxel followed by surgery in a nonrandomized phase II trial. Radiotherapy was administered in the event of progressive disease, positive margins, or persistent N2 disease. The regimen was well tolerated with no major nonhematologic toxicities. The response rate was 73.5% with induction therapy and 55% of patients underwent complete resection. Thirty-five percent of patients had complete mediastinal clearance at surgery. Median survival was 23 months.

The European Organization for Research and Treatment of Cancer (EORTC) 08941 study was a phase III trial evaluating outcomes in pathologically documented N2 NSCLC randomized to surgery or radiation therapy following partial response to platinum-based induction chemotherapy [23]. Three phase II feasibility studies evaluating different induction chemotherapy doublets were embedded within the trial design. In the first study (EORTC 08955), cisplatin and gemcitabine was given for three cycles to 47 patients. Thirty-three patients had an objective response, with 71% of the 17 patients undergoing surgical resection having complete resection. Median survival was reported for the entire patient population (inclusive of patients undergoing surgical resection and radiotherapy), and was 18.9 months [24]. In the second study (EORTC 08958),

Table 2
Induction chemotherapy trials with third generation agents

Primary author	Phase	Disease stage	No. of patients	Regimen	Objective response rate	Median survival	Survival with N2 downstaging
Betticher [21]	II	IIIA	90	CT × 3 → S (Adjuvant RT in 33 pts)	66%	27.6 mo	3-y Surv: 61% vs 11%
De Marinis [22]	II	IIIA	49	CGP × 3 →S	73.5%	23 mo 1-y Surv: 85%	—
Van Zandwijk (EORTC 08955) [24]	II	IIIA	47	CG × 3 →S vs RT	70%	18.9 mo Est 1-y Surv: 69%	—
O'Brien (EORTC 08958) [25]	II	IIIA	52	CaP × 3 →S vs RT	64%	20.5 mo Est 1-y Surv: 68.5%	—
Biesma (EORTC 08984) [26]	II	IIIA	46	CT × 3 →S vs RT	39%	16.7 mo 1-Y Surv: 64.6%	—
Cappuzzo [27]	II	IIIA-IIIB	129	CG × 4 →S or RT	62%	19.4 mo 1-Y Surv: 74%	—
Garrido [28]	II	IIIA-IIIB	136	CGT × 3 →S	56%	15.9 mo 5-y Surv: 21%	—

Abbreviations: Ca, carboplatin; C, cisplatin; Est, estimated; G, gemcitabine; Mo, months; P, paclitaxel; Pts, patients; RT, radiation; S, surgery; T, docetaxel; 3-y Surv, 3-year survival.

52 patients received induction therapy with three cycles of carboplatin and paclitaxel. Sixty-four percent had an objective response. Twelve of 15 patients randomized to the surgery arm underwent resection, although only 2 patients underwent complete resection. Median survival for all 52 patients was 20.5 months [25]. In the third trial (EORTC 08984), 46 patients received three cycles of cisplatin and docetaxel with 45% of patients showing an objective response. Median survival was reported as 15.8 months [26]. The conclusions of all three studies were that preoperative chemotherapy is feasible and effective [24–26]. Full results of the EORTC 08941 study are discussed in a following section.

The Italian Lung Cancer Project Observational Study [27] treated 129 patients with clinically unresectable, bulky N2, stage IIIA or IIIB NSCLC with four cycles of gemcitabine and cisplatin. Patients who responded to therapy would be considered for surgical resection, whereas patients with stable disease would receive definitive radiotherapy (60 Gy). Sixty-two percent of patients achieved a partial response, with 40 patients (31%) subsequently considered candidates for surgical resection. Complete resection was obtained in 38 patients (21 patients with stage IIIA tumors and 17 with stage IIIB tumors) for a resectability rate of 29%. Pathologic complete response was seen in two patients. Seventy patients went on to receive definitive radiotherapy. Major hematologic toxicities included grades 3 and 4 thrombocytopenia (27%), neutropenia (19%), and anemia (3%). Median survival was 19.4 months and the 1-year survival rate was 74%. The authors concluded that the combination of cisplatin and gemcitabine offered clinical activity as well as an acceptable toxicity profile, supporting ongoing investigation in randomized clinical trials.

A study conducted by the Spanish Lung Cancer Group (S9901) [28] looked at the combination of cisplatin, gemcitabine, and docetaxel administered for three cycles, followed by surgical resection, in 136 patients with pN2 disease or T4N0-1 NSCLC. Sixty-nine patients were stage IIIA with N2 involvement. Of 129 patients assessable, the response rate was 56%. Ninety patients (68.9%) underwent subsequent resection. Of the stage IIIA patients, 72% (33 of 46) underwent complete resection. Median survival for the entire group was 15.9 months, and 5-year survival was 21%. Survival in patients with stage IIIA (N2) disease did not differ from stage IIIB disease (15.6 versus 16.8 months). Of the 33 patients with stage IIIA disease able to undergo complete resection, median survival was 36.9 months, and 3- and 5-year survival rates were 50.2% and 31.6%, respectively.

These trials taken collectively show the feasibility and potential benefit of neoadjuvant therapy in stage IIIA (N2) disease with more modern chemotherapeutic combinations. Large-scale phase III survival data with these combinations in the neoadjuvant setting, however, are lacking. Conclusive proof of survival benefit with neoadjuvant chemotherapy alone is hampered by the small sample sizes in the phase III trials evaluating survival, as well as the use of older chemotherapeutic combinations. The optimal chemotherapeutic combination and duration of neoadjuvant treatment thus has yet to be defined.

Induction chemoradiotherapy

Given that concurrent chemoradiation is superior to sequential therapy in the definitive management of unresectable locally advanced NSCLC [29,30], a combined-modality approach has been investigated in the neoadjuvant setting for potentially resectable locally advanced NSCLC. Results of trials evaluating induction chemoradiotherapy are summarized in Table 3.

The phase II Southwest Oncology Group (SWOG) 8805 study was one of the first trials looking at induction chemoradiotherapy. This study included stage IIIA and IIIB tumors (bulky N2 and N3 nodal involvement and T4 disease) deemed initially unresectable. Patients received two cycles of cisplatin and etoposide and concurrent thoracic radiation to 45 Gy. Patients underwent surgical resection via thoracotomy in the absence of progressive disease. Patients with complete resections, negative mediastinal nodes and negative surgical margins received no further therapy. Patients with unresectable disease, incomplete resections, or positive mediastinal nodal involvement underwent further chemotherapy with two cycles of cisplatin and etoposide concurrently with radiation to a total dose of 59 Gy. Of 126 eligible patients, 82 had N2 disease. The objective response rate for the entire study group was 59%, while 29% had stable disease. No difference in response patterns was seen between stage IIIA and IIIB disease. One hundred seven patients (85%) were eligible for thoracotomy after induction [31].

Table 3
Induction chemoradiotherapy trials

Primary author	Phase	Disease stage	No. Pts	Regimen	ORR	Survival	*P* value	TRM	Survival with N2 downstaging
Albain (SWOG 8805) [31]	II	IIIA-IIIB	126	CE × 2 + RT (45 Gy) → S	59%	Med Surv: IIIA: 13 mo; IIIB: 17 mo; 3-Y S: IIIA: 27%; IIIB: 24%	.81	10%	Med Surv: 30 mo (N0) vs 9 mo (N1-3); P = .003
Albain (Intergroup 0139) [32]	III	IIIA	429	CE × 2 + RT (45 Gy) → S Vs RT (61 Gy); → CE × 2	NR	OS: S: 23.6 mo; RT: 22.2 mo 5-y S: S: 27.2% RT: 20.3%	0.24	S: 7.9% (26% with pneumonec-tomy) RT: 2.1%	34 mo vs 26 mo (P = NR) 5-y S: 41% (N0) vs 24% (N1-3) vs 8% (No Surgery); *P* < .0001
Katatyama [34]	II	IIIA-IIIB	22	CT × 4 + RT (40-60 Gy) → S	73%	Est 3-y S: 66%	—	—	—
Eberhardt [35]	II	IIIA-IIIB	64	CP × 3 →CE + RT (45 Gy) → S	84%	Med Surv: 25 mo 4-y S: 30%	—	—	—

Abbreviations: C, cisplatin; E, etoposide; Est, estimated; Med Surv, median survival; Mo, months; NR, not reported; ORR, overall response rate; OS, overall survival; P, paclitaxel; Pts, patients; RT, radiation; S, surgery; T, docetaxel; TRM, treatment-related mortality; 3-y S, 3-year survival.

Treatment-related mortality was reported as 10%. Two patients died during induction (from pseudomembranous colitis and idiopathic thrombocytopenic purpura–like syndrome, respectively). Eight deaths occurred during the postoperative period, with six of these occurring in patients undergoing pneumonectomies. The causes of death included adult respiratory distress syndrome (ARDS) and pulmonary embolus (two patients each), ARDS and pseudomonal sepsis, ARDS with multiple microemboli, unstable hemodynamics, and respiratory failure (one event each). Three more deaths occurred during boost chemoradiotherapy (pneumonia in two events; pulmonary embolus with pneumonitis, one event). Three-year overall survival for the entire eligible population was 27%. No difference in survival was noted between stage IIIA or IIIB tumors, although the study was not powered to detect a difference in survival between these groups (median survival 13 versus 17 months, respectively; $P = .81$). Pathologic clearance of the mediastinum predicted a more favorable outcome for N2 disease than did persistent N2 involvement (median survival 30 months versus 9 months, respectively; $P = .003$). Given the significant postoperative mortality, this study raised the question of the appropriateness of surgical resection if induction therapy has cleared the mediastinum, and acknowledged that this issue would need to be explored further in the context of a randomized trial [31].

The results and observations from the SWOG 8805 trial led to the North American Intergroup 0139 randomized phase III trial involving 429 patients with stage IIIA tumors with N2 involvement. The regimen was based on the SWOG 8805 trial, with patients receiving induction cisplatin and etoposide concurrently with 45 Gy of radiation, followed by either surgical resection or definitive radiation to a total dose of 61 Gy. After completion of either resection or definitive radiation, patients received two cycles of consolidation cisplatin and etoposide [32].

No deaths occurred during induction therapy. Treatment-related mortality was 7.9% in the surgery arm and 2.1% in the chemoradiotherapy arm. The majority of the deaths in the surgery arm were in patients undergoing pneumonectomies (14 deaths with 26% mortality), especially right-sided pneumonectomy (11 deaths). Overall survival was similar (23.6 months with surgery versus 22.2 months with chemoradiation; $P = .24$), but progression-free survival favored the surgery group (12.8 versus 10.5 months, respectively; $P = .017$). In an exploratory subset analysis, patients undergoing lobectomy had a survival advantage over those undergoing definitive chemoradiotherapy (median survival 34 versus 22 months; $P = .002$). Patients with pathologic downstaging to N0 status demonstrated a survival benefit compared with those patients with persistent nodal involvement (N1–N3 disease, or nodal involvement "unknown") at the time of surgery, and with patients who did not undergo surgical resection (5-year survival 41% versus 24% versus 8%, respectively; $P < .0001$). A trend toward worse overall survival was noted when those undergoing pneumonectomy were compared with those undergoing chemoradiotherapy alone (median survival 19 months versus 29 months, $P =$ NS). These results have led to the consideration of pneumonectomy as a relative contraindication for surgical resection in patients with locally advanced NSCLC and N2 involvement [32].

Uy and colleagues [33] published a retrospective single-institution series of 40 patients who underwent induction chemoradiation followed by surgical resection and consolidation chemotherapy similar to the Intergroup 0139 trial (16 patients in this series had been included on the surgical arm of the Intergroup 0139 trial). All the patients had biopsy-proven NSCLC with N2 involvement. Overall response rate was 67.5%. Overall and disease- free survival for the entire group was 40.0 and 37.1 months, respectively. Overall 3-year survival was 51.7%. The overall operative mortality was 7.5%. Of the 29 patients undergoing lobectomy, postoperative mortality was 0%; postoperative mortality for patients undergoing pneumonectomy was 27%. While the results of a single-institution retrospective patient series cannot be directly compared with the results of a multicenter phase III trial, similarities in mortality among patients undergoing pneumonectomy after induction therapy further supports caution in this patient group. The results of this series additionally further supports the concept that in carefully selected patients, treatment in accordance to the Intergroup 0139 induction protocol may result in improved survival with longer overall and disease-free survival.

Katayama and associates [34] conducted a feasibility study evaluating cisplatin and docetaxel administered on days 1, 8, 29, and 36 with concurrent radiotherapy of 40 to 60 Gy followed by surgery in 22 patients with stage IIIA (n = 14) and

IIIB (n = 8) disease. The objective response rate was 73%. Twenty patients (91%) underwent surgery, with complete resection occurring in 19 patients (86%). There were no treatment-related deaths during induction therapy or after surgery. The calculated 3-year overall and progression-free survival rates were 66% and 61%. Pathologic downstaging and complete response were demonstrated in 14 (64%) and 5 (23%) patients, respectively, suggesting that local control can be achieved with concurrent chemoradiotherapy as induction therapy.

Whereas Katayama and colleagues [34] used standard fractionated radiotherapy, Eberhardt and colleagues [35] treated 64 patients with inoperable stage IIIA and IIIB disease with three 21-day cycles of cisplatin and paclitaxel, followed by cisplatin and etoposide concurrent with hyperfractionated radiotherapy (45 Gy, 1.5 Gy twice daily). Overall response rate was 84% (54/64 patients). Thirty-six patients (56%) underwent thoracotomy, with 32 undergoing complete resection. Overall median survival was 25 months, and 36 months for those patients who had a complete resection. Four-year overall survival was 30%, and 49% in those patients who had complete resections.

These studies suggest that induction chemotherapy and radiotherapy followed by surgery may be feasible, although a direct comparison of neoadjuvant chemotherapy versus chemoradiotherapy followed by surgical resection is lacking. Clearance of the mediastinum appears to be associated with better outcomes. The ideal combination of chemotherapy and radiotherapy for induction remains to be determined.

Role of surgery

The appropriate selection of patients for surgery following neoadjuvant therapy continues to be a challenge for all specialists who deal with locally advanced NSCLC. Concern about increased morbidity and mortality of resection following induction therapy emphasizes the importance of selecting patients who may benefit from surgical intervention [32,33]. Accurate restaging is essential to identify disease refractory to induction therapy in order to reduce the operative risk of surgery in patients who may not benefit.

For those showing a response to induction, surgical resection has a role in multimodality therapy. As demonstrated in the SAKK study and in the SWOG 8805 trial, pathologic downstaging with mediastinal clearance of disease strongly predicted survival [21,31]. The Intergroup 0139 study noted a survival benefit for the 76 patients with pathologic downstaging to N0 status compared with patients with persistent nodal disease (88 patients) and those who did not undergo surgery (38 patients), with median survival of 34 months with N0, 26 months with N1–N3 disease, and 8 months without surgery ($P < .0001$) [32].

Bueno and colleagues [36] published a retrospective single-institution series exploring the predictive value of nodal status at resection in regard to long-term outcomes for patients with stage IIIA N2 NSCLC. One hundred and three patient charts were reviewed. A mix of different neoadjuvant therapies was used, including 76 patients receiving platinum-based chemotherapy, 18 patients receiving single-modality thoracic radiation, and 9 patients receiving combination chemoradiation. Of 29 patients downstaged to pathologic N0 disease following induction therapy, survival was superior compared with the 74 patients with residual nodal disease at surgery (49 with persistent N2 disease). Median survival was 21.3 months for N0 disease versus 15.9 months with residual nodal disease, 5-year survival was 35.8% versus 9%, respectively ($P = .023$).

In a single institutional review from France, Barlési and associates [37] reported outcomes of 71 patients with stage IIIA N2 NSCLC who had surgery following neoadjuvant treatment. The patients received two to four cycles of platinum in combination with vinorelbine (33 patients), etoposide (18 patients), paclitaxel (9 patients), gemcitabine (9 patients), or ifosamide and mitomycin (2 patients). Fifteen patients received concurrent thoracic radiotherapy with induction chemotherapy (20 to 45 Gy). The response rate to neoadjuvant therapy was 50.7%. Of 66 patients who underwent surgical resection, 61 had complete resection, and 9 patients demonstrated pathologic complete response. Forty-four percent underwent lobectomy and 42% either had a right or left pneumonectomy, with the remainder having either bilobectomy, wedge resection, or exploratory thoracotomy without full resection. Operative mortality was 4.2%, with operative morbidity of 29%. Median survival was 17 months with 3- and 5-year survival being 24% and 13%, respectively. Persistent disease in mediastinal lymph nodes at the time of surgical resection was associated with poor outcome (relative risk of death 2.7; $P = .002$), while responders to treatment and those achieving N0 status had a favorable outcome (5-year survival 25.5% for those with mediastinal clearance and 0% survival with incomplete mediastinal clearance, $P = .01$).

Other series have looked at the outcome specifically of pneumonectomies following induction therapy. Doddoli and colleagues [38] evaluated 100 pneumonectomies performed after induction therapy in a single-institution series (79 in patients with N2 disease). All patients received two to four cycles of a platinum-based doublet; in combination with vinorelbine in 46 patients, etoposide in 25 patients, gemcitabine in 15 patients, and paclitaxel in 14 patients. Thirty patients were treated with concurrent thoracic radiotherapy (30 to 45 Gy). The response rates to induction therapy were not reported. Ninety-four patients had complete resection, with eight patients demonstrating pathologic complete response. The 30- and 90-day mortalities were 12% and 21%, respectively. Postoperative cardiovascular and respiratory events were predictive of both 30- and 90-day mortality, with age greater than 60 years and need for transfusion additionally predictive of 90-day mortality. Right- or left-sided pneumonectomy did not predict for postoperative mortality in this series. The estimated 5-year overall survival was 19.8%. The authors concluded that pneumonectomy following induction therapy is a high-risk procedure, with uncertain curative benefit over alternative procedures.

Allen and associates [39] reported outcomes of 73 pneumonectomies following neoadjuvant therapy performed at the Dana-Farber Cancer Institute. Neoadjuvant therapy consisted of concurrent chemoradiotherapy in 69 patients, and single-modality radiation in the remaining 4 patients (median dose of radiation 54 Gy in all patients). Fifty-one percent of patients had stage IIIA disease. Left pneumonectomy was performed in 45 patients, with 28 patients undergoing right pneumonectomy. Response rates, complete resection, and occurrence of persistent lymph node involvement were not reported. The 30- and 100-day mortality rates were 6% and 10%, respectively. Median survival was 23 months, with 2-year survival 49%. Despite the fact that both of these series reported better survival than those reported in the Intergroup 0139 trial, as single-institution series there is no ability to compare with a statistically powered multi-institutional randomized phase III trial. The authors however do raise the question of greater feasibility of pneumonectomy following neoadjuvant therapy when performed in high-volume experienced institutions.

The EORTC study 08941 enrolled 579 patients with cytologically or histologically proven unresectable stage IIIA (N2) NSCLC to undergo either surgery or radiation after induction chemotherapy [23]. Patients received three cycles of platinum-based chemotherapy. Owing to low accrual, the study was prematurely closed, with 332 of a planned 358 patients randomized. Overall response was 61% with induction therapy, and 57% of patients with a clinical response were subsequently randomized to surgical resection or definitive radiotherapy. Of the 165 patients randomized to radiotherapy, 93% were treated. Of the 167 patients randomized to resection, 92% underwent surgery, with 47% undergoing pneumonectomy. Fifty percent had an R0 resection, and pathologic complete response was demonstrated in 5%. Sixty-two patients (40%) received postoperative radiation. No significant difference was detected between the two arms in terms of either median survival or 5-year survival (median survival 17.5 months with surgery versus 16.4 months with radiation, 5-year survival 14% versus 15.7%, respectively; P = NS). Progression-free survival rates were similar between the groups (11.3 months versus 9 months; P = NS). In an unplanned subgroup analysis, 5-year survival favored mediastinal downstaging to N0 or N1 status compared with persistent N2 disease at the time of resection (29% versus 7%, respectively; $P < .001$), as well as complete resection versus incomplete resection (5-year survival 27% versus 7%; $P < .001$). Patients who underwent lobectomy or bilobectomy had better outcomes than those who had pneumonectomies (5-year survival 27% versus 12%, respectively; $P = .009$). The authors concluded that for patients with stage IIIA N2 NSCLC, surgery does not improve survival compared with definitive radiation, and that because of the lower morbidity and mortality, radiation should be the preferred definitive locoregional therapy for N2 disease [23].

Further randomized studies will be needed to help determine the optimal selection of patients most likely to benefit from surgery following induction therapy for NSCLC with N2 disease. The question still remains whether patients who have mediastinal clearance should undergo surgical resection considering the associated risks of morbidity and mortality. Persistent mediastinal disease has now been shown to correlate with poor outcomes in multiple studies [21,30,31,35,36]. Lobectomy appears to be a feasible procedure following induction chemotherapy and radiotherapy [33,39]. Pneumonectomies can have a high incidence of postoperative mortality based on both individual institutional and phase III trial experience, which may eliminate poor operative candidates should a pneumonectomy be required for complete resection [30–32]. Patients able to undergo a complete resection may have improved overall and median survival following induction therapy for stage IIIA NSCLC [34,39].

Induction therapy with molecularly targeted agents

A number of molecularly targeted agents have now been shown to prolong life for patients with NSCLC in the setting of advanced disease. These include monoclonal antibodies as well as a small molecule tyrosine kinase inhibitor. A large number of new targeted agents are in various stages of testing and clinical development. Bevacizumab, a monoclonal antibody targeted against vascular endothelial growth factor (VEGF), has been shown to prolong survival in combination with chemotherapy for patients with advanced and metastatic nonsquamous NSCLC [40]. Cetuximab, a monoclonal antibody targeted against the epidermal growth factor receptor (EGFR), prolongs survival in combination with chemotherapy for patients with NSCLC when compared with chemotherapy alone, in addition to prolonging survival for patients with advanced colorectal cancers and squamous cell carcinomas of the head and neck [41–43]. Erlotinib is a small molecule EGFR tyrosine kinase inhibitor that prolongs survival for patients with recurrent advanced or metastatic NSCLC [44].

The favorable toxicity profile of the targeted agents relative to standard chemotherapy offers the promise of improved tolerance to therapy coupled with the hope of improving efficacy. Based on the survival gains demonstrated in advanced disease, evaluation is now ongoing with targeted agents in earlier-stage disease. Large trials are lacking, but early-phase studies are discussed in the following sections.

Bevacizumab

Rizvi and colleagues [45] have reported preliminary findings of an ongoing study investigating the feasibility of incorporating bevacizumab into the neoadjuvant and adjuvant therapy of resectable NSCLC (stages IB–IIIA). In a two-cohort model, patients with adenocarcinoma received a single dose of bevacizumab, followed by one cycle of cisplatin and docetaxel, then two cycles of chemotherapy and bevacizumab in combination, followed by surgical resection. Patients with squamous cell lung cancer received neoadjuvant cisplatin and docetaxel in the second cohort. Both cohorts then underwent surgical resection, followed by 1 year of adjuvant bevacizumab. Initial results of the first 19 of 70 planned patients included 11 patients treated in the first cohort (9 with stage IIIA NSCLC). After the initial dose of single-agent bevacizumab, 6 of the 11 patients had greater than 10% tumor reduction. After bevacizumab and chemotherapy, 6 of 10 patients showed partial response. Six of 10 patients went on to have complete resections. One patient developed preoperative hemoptysis, and one patient developed a postoperative gastrointestinal bleed. No other bevacizumab-related operative complications were observed. Of the eight patients in the second cohort, all have undergone complete resection. Treatment and accrual to this study are ongoing, but preliminary results demonstrate tolerability in the preoperative setting.

Cetuximab

Coate and associates [46] have reported preliminary results of a phase II pilot study evaluating the combination of cetuximab with cisplatin and gemcitabine as neoadjuvant therapy for patients with resectable stage IB through IIIA NSCLC. Of 16 patients enrolled in the ongoing study, 9 had stage IIIA disease. Response rate for all patients enrolled was 37.5%. Further data are awaited at the time of completion of accrual.

Erlotinib

Erlotinib is currently being investigated in the neoadjuvant setting for NSCLC in several different ongoing trials. The Surgery for Early Lung Cancer with Preoperative Erlotinib (SELECT) study is a phase II trial evaluating single-agent erlotinib before surgical resection for patients with stage I and II NSCLC. A similar phase II trial of stage I to IIIA NSCLC conducted by the Eastern Cooperative Oncology Group has now stopped accruing patients. In stage III disease, a phase I/II study testing the combination of erlotinib with carboplatin and paclitaxel with accelerated hyperfractionated radiation, followed by surgical resection and maintenance erlotinib, is currently accruing patients [47].

Other targeted agents

Vandetanib, a tyrosine kinase inhibitor targeting both the VEGF receptor and EGFR, is currently undergoing evaluation in a phase II trial in the neoadjuvant setting. Patients with resectable stage I to III (excluding patients with N2 disease) NSCLC receive vandetanib in combination with carboplatin and paclitaxel for up to three cycles before surgical resection [47].

Summary

The optimal treatment for stage IIIA (N2) NSCLC remains controversial. Numerous studies with induction chemotherapy or chemoradiotherapy show that both approaches in the neoadjuvant setting are feasible. Outcomes following induction therapy have been associated with mediastinal nodal response, with residual mediastinal involvement a negative predictor of survival. Appropriate selection of patients to undergo resection following induction therapy is critical. Lobectomy may be safely performed following induction therapy while pneumonectomy may carry a high and possibly unacceptable rate of perioperative mortality.

Combined modality therapy has increased the overall survival of patients with stage III NSCLC. Future trials looking at different induction regimens with or without radiotherapy and with or without surgery may help identify the ideal treatment for this heterogeneous disease stage. The SAKK-16/00 study is an ongoing phase III European trial randomizing patients with stage IIIA NSCLC to receive neoadjuvant chemotherapy with three cycles of docetaxel and cisplatin followed by radiation and then surgical resection, or to chemotherapy with the same regimen followed by surgery alone [47].

Other ongoing trials include investigations of novel chemotherapeutic combinations, such as cisplatin with pemetrexed, in the phase II setting. The RTOG 0229 phase II study is evaluating neoadjuvant paclitaxel and carboplatin concurrently with radiation therapy, followed by surgery and consolidation chemotherapy with paclitaxel and carboplatin for stage III NSCLC. The combination of neoadjuvant docetaxel, carboplatin, and radiation therapy followed by surgical resection for stage III NSCLC is also currently being investigated in a phase II trial [47].

The future of treatment for stage III NSCLC may lie in the outcome of trials investigating molecularly targeted agents, such as EGFR inhibitors, anti-angiogenic agents, or multitargeted agents. Optimal incorporation into the multimodality approach required of locally advanced N2 NSCLC will require careful investigation. The results from these trials are eagerly awaited.

References

[1] National Cancer Institute. Surveilance, epidemiologic, and end results public use data 2007. Available at: http://seer.cancer.gov. Accessed July 14, 2008.
[2] Mountain CF. Revisions in the international system for staging lung cancer. Chest 1997;111:1710–7.
[3] Jemal A, Siegel R, Ward E, et al. Cancer statistics, 2007. CA Cancer J Clin 2007;57:43–66.
[4] DeCamp MM Jr, Ashiku S, Thurer R. The role of surgery in N2 non-small cell lung cancer. Clin Cancer Res 2005;11:5033s–7s.
[5] Rami-Porta R, Ball D, Crowley J, et al. The IASLC lung cancer staging project: proposals for the revision of the T descriptors in the forthcoming (seventh) edition of the TNM classification for lung cancer. J Thorac Oncol 2007;2:593–602.
[6] Rusch VW, Crowley J, Giroux DJ, et al. The IASLC lung cancer staging project: proposals for the revision of the N descriptors in the forthcoming seventh edition of the TNM classification for lung cancer. J Thorac Oncol 2007;2:603–12.
[7] Postmus PE, Brambilla E, Chansky K, et al. The IASLC lung cancer staging project: proposals for revision of the M descriptors in the forthcoming (seventh) edition of the TNM classification of lung cancer. J Thorac Oncol 2007;2:686–93.
[8] Prenzel KL, Mönig SP, Sinning JM, et al. Lymph node size and metastatic infiltration in non-small cell lung cancer. Chest 2003;123:463–7.
[9] Choi YS, Shim YM, Kim J, et al. Mediastinoscopy in patients with clinical stage I non-small cell lung cancer. Ann Thorac Surg 2003;75:364–6.
[10] Toloza EM, Harpole L, McCrory DC. Noninvasive staging of non-small cell lung cancer: a review of the current evidence. Chest 2003;123:137S–46S.
[11] Birim O, Kappetein AP, Stijnen T, et al. Meta-analysis of positron emission tomographic and computed tomographic imaging in detecting mediastinal lymph node metastases in nonsmall cell lung cancer. Ann Thorac Surg 2005;79:375–82.
[12] Lardinois D, Weder W, Hany TF, et al. Staging of non-small-cell lung cancer with integrated positron-emission tomography and computed tomography. N Engl J Med 2003;348:2500–7.

[13] Toloza EM, Harpole L, Detterbeck F, et al. Invasive staging of non-small cell lung cancer: a review of the current evidence. Chest 2003;123:157S–66S.

[14] Meko J, Rusch VW. Neoadjuvant therapy and surgical resection for locally advanced non-small cell lung cancer. Semin Radiat Oncol 2000;10:324–32.

[15] Martini N, Kris MG, Flehinger BJ, et al. Preoperative chemotherapy for stage IIIa (N2) lung cancer: the Sloan-Kettering experience with 136 patients. Ann Thorac Surg 1993;55:1365–73 [discussion: 1373–4].

[16] Rosell R, Gómez-Codina J, Camps C, et al. A randomized trial comparing preoperative chemotherapy plus surgery with surgery alone in patients with non-small-cell lung cancer. N Engl J Med 1994;330:153–8.

[17] Rosell R, Gomez-Codina J, Camps C, et al. Preresectional chemotherapy in stage IIIA non-small-cell lung cancer: a 7-year assessment of a randomized controlled trial. Lung Cancer 1999;26:7–14.

[18] Roth JA, Fossella F, Komaki R, et al. A randomized trial comparing perioperative chemotherapy and surgery with surgery alone in resectable stage IIIA non-small-cell lung cancer. J Natl Cancer Inst 1994;86:673–80.

[19] Pass HI, Pogrebniak HW, Steinberg SM, et al. Randomized trial of neoadjuvant therapy for lung cancer: interim analysis. Ann Thorac Surg 1992;53: 992–8.

[20] Depierre A, Milleron B, Moro-Sibilot D, et al. Preoperative chemotherapy followed by surgery compared with primary surgery in resectable stage I (except T1N0), II, and IIIA non-small-cell lung cancer. J Clin Oncol 2002;20:247–53.

[21] Betticher DC, Hsu Schmitz SF, Tötsch M, et al. Mediastinal lymph node clearance after docetaxel-cisplatin neoadjuvant chemotherapy is prognostic of survival in patients with stage IIIA pN2 non-small-cell lung cancer: a multicenter phase II trial. J Clin Oncol 2003;21:1752–9.

[22] De Marinis F, Nelli F, Migliorino MR, et al. Gemcitabine, paclitaxel, and cisplatin as induction chemotherapy for patients with biopsy-proven Stage IIIA (N2) nonsmall cell lung carcinoma: a Phase II multicenter study. Cancer 2003;98:1707–15.

[23] van Meerbeeck JP, Kramer GW, van Schil PE, et al. Randomized controlled trial of resection versus radiotherapy after induction chemotherapy in stage IIIA-N2 non-small-cell lung cancer. J Natl Cancer Inst 2007;99:442–50.

[24] Van Zandwijk N, Smit EF, Kramer GW, et al. Gemcitabine and cisplatin as induction regimen for patients with biopsy-proven stage IIIA N2 non-small-cell lung cancer: a phase II study of the European Organization for Research and Treatment of Cancer Lung Cancer Cooperative Group (EORTC 08955). J Clin Oncol 2000;18:2658–64.

[25] O'Brien ME, Splinter T, Smit EF, et al. Carboplatin and paclitaxel (Taxol) as an induction regimen for patients with biopsy-proven stage IIIA N2 non-small cell lung cancer: an EORTC phase II study (EORTC 08958). Eur J Cancer 2003;39:1416–22.

[26] Biesma B, Manegold C, Smit HJ, et al. Docetaxel and cisplatin as induction chemotherapy in patients with pathologically-proven stage IIIA N2 non-small cell lung cancer: a phase II study of the European Organization for Research and Treatment of Cancer (EORTC 08984). Eur J Cancer 2006;42:1399–406.

[27] Cappuzzo F, Selvaggi G, Gregorc V, et al. Gemcitabine and cisplatin as induction chemotherapy for patients with unresectable Stage IIIA-bulky N2 and Stage IIIB nonsmall cell lung carcinoma: an Italian Lung Cancer Project Observational Study. Cancer 2003;98:128–34.

[28] Garrido P, González-Larriba JL, Insa A, et al. Long-term survival associated with complete resection after induction chemotherapy in stage IIIA (N2) and IIIB (T4N0-1) non small-cell lung cancer patients: the Spanish Lung Cancer Group Trial 9901. J Clin Oncol 2007;25:4736–42.

[29] Furuse K, Fukuoka M, Kawahara M, et al. Phase III study of concurrent versus sequential thoracic radiotherapy in combination with mitomycin, vindesine, and cisplatin in unresectable stage III non-small-cell lung cancer. J Clin Oncol 1999;17:2692–9.

[30] Curran WJ, Scott CB, Langer CJ, et al. Long-term benefit is observed in a phase III comparison of sequential vs concurrent chemo-radiation for patients with unresected stage III NSCLC: RTOG 9410 [abstract]. Proc Am Soc Clin Oncol 2003;22:2499.

[31] Albain KS, Rusch VW, Crowley JJ, et al. Concurrent cisplatin/etoposide plus chest radiotherapy followed by surgery for stages IIIA (N2) and IIIB non-small-cell lung cancer: mature results of Southwest Oncology Group phase II study 8805. J Clin Oncol 1995;13:1880–92.

[32] Albain KS, Swann RS, Rusch VW, et al. Phase III study of concurrent chemotherapy and radiotherapy (CT/RT) vs CT/RT followed by surgical resection for stage IIIA (pN2) non-small cell lung cancer (NSCLC): outcomes update of North American Intergroup 0139 (RTOG 9309). Proc Am Soc Clin Oncol 2005;23:7014 [abstract].

[33] Uy KL, Darling G, Xu W, et al. Improved results of induction chemoradiation before surgical intervention for selected patients with stage IIIA-N2 non-small cell lung cancer. J Thorac Cardiovasc Surg 2007;134:188–93.

[34] Katayama H, Ueoka H, Kiura K, et al. Preoperative concurrent chemoradiotherapy with cisplatin and docetaxel in patients with locally advanced non-small-cell lung cancer. Br J Cancer 2004;90:979–84.

[35] Eberhardt W, Le Pechoux C, Gauler T. Multicenter German/French phase II trial of induction chemotherapy (CTx) followed by hyperfractionated accelerated thoracic radiotherapy with CTx +/- surgery in locally advanced inoperable non-small cell lung cancer stage III patients: mature results of a novel

induction CTx regimen. Lung Cancer 2004;46: S40–41 [abstract].

[36] Bueno R, Richards WG, Swanson SJ, et al. Nodal stage after induction therapy for stage IIIA lung cancer determines patient survival. Ann Thorac Surg 2000;70:1826–31.

[37] Barlési F, Doddoli C, Chetaille B, et al. Survival and postoperative complication in daily practice after neoadjuvant therapy in resectable stage IIIA-N2 non-small cell lung cancer. Interact Cardiovasc Thorac Surg 2003;2:558–62.

[38] Doddoli C, Barlesi F, Trousse D, et al. One hundred consecutive pneumonectomies after induction therapy for non-small cell lung cancer: an uncertain balance between risks and benefits. J Thorac Cardiovasc Surg 2005;130:416–25.

[39] Allen AM, Mentzer SJ, Yeap BY, et al. Pneumonectomy after chemoradiation: the Dana-Farber Cancer Institute/Brigham and Women's Hospital experience. Cancer 2008;112:1106–13.

[40] Sandler AB, Gray R, Perry MC, et al. Paclitaxel-carboplatin alone or with bevacizumab for non-small-cell lung cancer. N Engl J Med 2006;355:2542–50.

[41] Pirker R, Szczesna A, von Pawel J, et al. FLEX: a randomized, multicenter, phase III study of cetuximab in combination with cisplatin/vinorelbine versus CV alone in the first-line treatment of patients with advanced non-small cell lung cancer. Proc Am Soc Clin Oncol 2008;26:3 [abstract].

[42] Sobrero AF, Maurel J, Fehrenbacher L, et al. EPIC: phase III trial of cetuximab plus irinotecan after fluoropyrimidine and oxaliplatin failure in patients with metastatic colorectal cancer. J Clin Oncol 2008;26:2311–9.

[43] Vermorken J, Mesia R, Vega V, et al. Cetuximab extends survival of patients with recurrent or metastatic SCCHN when added to first line platinum based therapy-Results of a randomized phase III (Extreme) study. Proc Am Soc Clin Oncol 2007;25: 6091 [abstract].

[44] Shepherd FA, Pereira JR, Ciuleanu T, et al. Erlotinib in previously treated non-small-cell lung cancer. N Engl J Med 2005;353:123–32.

[45] Rizvi NA, Rusch V, Zhao B, et al. Single agent bevacizumab and bevacizumab in combination with docetaxel and cisplatin as induction therapy for resectable IB-IIIA non-small cell lung cancer. Proc Am Soc Clin Oncol 2007;25:18045 [abstract].

[46] Coate LE, Gately K, Barr M, et al. Phase II pilot study of neoadjuvant cetuximab in combination with cisplatin and gemcitabine in patients with resectable IB-IIIA non small cell lung cancer. Proc Am Soc Clin Oncol 2006;24:17107 [abstract].

[47] Available at: www.clinicaltrials.gov.

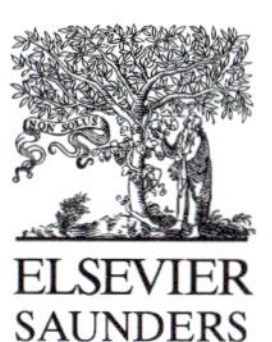
ELSEVIER
SAUNDERS

Thorac Surg Clin 18 (2008) 417–421

THORACIC
SURGERY
CLINICS

Restaging After Neo-Adjuvant Chemoradiotherapy for N2 Non–Small Cell Lung Cancer

Robert J. Cerfolio, MD, FACS, FCCP[a,*], Ayesha S. Bryant, MSPH, MD[b]

[a]*Section of Thoracic Surgery, Division of Cardiothoracic Surgery, Department of Surgery, University of Alabama at Birmingham, 703 19th Street S, ZRB 739, Birmingham, AL 35294, USA*

[b]*Division of Cardiothoracic Surgery, Department of Surgery and Department of Epidemiology, University of Alabama at Birmingham School of Public Health, Birmingham, AL, USA*

The treatment of non–small-cell lung cancer (NSCLC) depends on the stage. In 2004, 170,000 Americans were diagnosed with NSCLC, and almost one in five patients presented with N2 or stage IIIA disease [1]. Therefore, N2 disease is common. As described in the previous articles in this issue, there are many different types of N2 disease and numerous ways to diagnose and treat it [2]. In this article we reserve our comments to metastatic lymph nodes that have been described previously by us [3] and others as "mobile" or "nonfixed" or "nonbulky" N2 disease. This is a different type of N2 disease and one that may benefit from surgical resection after the use of preoperative chemoradiotherapy [4,5]. The decision as to how to treat the different types of N2 disease should be made before commencing neoadjuvant therapy and is why we favor using "curative doses" of preoperative radiation of 60 Gy or higher and not the more commonly used 45 Gy.

Recent studies have shown that patients who are down-staged via neoadjuvant therapy and undergo resection have a significant increased 5-year survival rate (as high as 40%–50%) [3,6–8] when compared with patients who have residual N2 disease [9]. The identification of patients who are N2 negative after the completion of their neoadjuvant therapy is a critical component of proper patient selection for thoracotomy. Some may even argue that it is a necessary step before resection. In this article we review the best ways to restage patients with N2 disease after they have completed their neoadjuvant therapy.

Preoperative staging, N2

The restaging of patients with N2 disease is only as good as the initial staging. Too often patients are sent to surgeons after their preoperative radiation and chemotherapy have started or even finished but their true staged has not been assessed. Recall pathologic stage is defined as the "stage after the patient has undergone video-assisted thoracoscopic surgery (VATS) or thoracotomy with intent for complete resection and tumor removal," and biopsies of lymph nodes via endoscopic ultrasound (EUS), endobronchial ultrasound (EBUS), VATS, or even thoracotomy are still referred to as clinical stage and not true pathologic stage. Because this concept and terminology is often confusing, we refer to the stage that is determined after procedures that biopsy mediastinal N2 lymph nodes as "the clinical stage after mediastinal lymph node biopsies [3]."Initial staging, much like repeat staging, must use tissue biopsies of lymph nodes to prove N2 disease and rule out M1 disease. The targets that should be biopsied are suggested by the integrated positron emission tomography (PET)/CT and CT scans. The continued practice of assuming that lymph nodes are positive because they are "really hot on PET scan" or "really big on CT scan" is absolutely wrong. It is unacceptable and provides poor care.

* Corresponding author.
E-mail address: rcerfolio@uab.edu (R.J. Cerfolio).

1547-4127/08/$ - see front matter
doi:10.1016/j.thorsurg.2008.08.002

We and others recommend initial staging that features integrated PET/CT scans and CT scan using intravenous contrast with 5-mm columinated cuts. Only the brain and the bone can be deemed as containing cancer—or not—without undergoing a biopsy. The best scan for those patients is an MRI that is unequivocal and consistent with the patients' clinical picture and other blood chemistries. All other suspicious targets suggested by either PET/CT or by CT must be biopsied, and a negative biopsy result does not necessarily confirm benignancy. Patients with highly suspicious N2 or N3 targets may require more than one biopsy (ie, not only an EBUS or EUS with fine needle aspiration [FNA] but also mediastinoscopy) to ensure the presence or absence of N2 or N3 disease before pulmonary resection.

Sometimes a VATS or open thoracotomy is warranted if clinical suspicion is high and the other test results are negative. The new techniques for mediastinal lymph node biopsies that are available (including video mediastinoscopy, EBUS, and EUS-FNA) should be used. EUS-FNA is the best minimally invasive test to stage the posterior mediastinum (lymph node stations 7, 8, and 9); EBUS and mediastinoscopy are better for the middle mediastinum. VATS and open thoracotomy can assess all of the stations. We recently described left VATS as an effective minimally invasive technique to biopsy the number 5 and 6 lymph nodes. If a patient is strongly suspected to have N2 disease after PET/CT or CT scan and results of EBUS or EUS are negative, mediastinoscopy still must be performed to ensure that these less invasive test results are not false negative, especially if the endosonographer is still on the ascent of his or her learning curve.

Some thoracic surgeons consistently perform mediastinoscopy before any pulmonary resection for NSCLC regardless of the size of the primary tumor or its location. We have shown in a prospective study that mediastinoscopy and EUS-FNA find unsuspected or nonimaged N2 disease in only 2.9% and 3.7% of patients with NSCLC who are staged as N0 after both PET and CT; thus we do not recommend their routine use [10]. Myers and associates also demonstrated similar data [11]. The advantage of preoperative chemotherapy or chemoradiotherapy before pulmonary resection as compared with resection followed by adjuvant chemotherapy is unknown for patients with this type of unsuspected N2 disease. We and others have labeled this type of N2 disease "radiographically silent," "unsuspected," "microscopic," or—even more specifically—"CT and PET negative." The best treatment of these patients presents another controversy that is outside the scope of this article [2]. In another study, we showed that patients who undergo complete resection and have unsuspected N2 disease after integrated PET/CT and 5-mm cut-contrasted CT scans have an overall 5-year survival rate of 37%.

Once nonbulky or mobile N2 disease is diagnosed and higher stage disease (bulky N2 or N3 and M1) is ruled out, then preoperative chemotherapy and radiotherapy should be administered. We prefer to use 60 Gy and, more recently, even higher doses (up to 72 Gy). The reason we prefer this regimen has been well described [12]. A brief summary of this concept is provided. A higher amount of radiotherapy affords patients the opportunity to maximize their medical therapy in case they do not undergo resection after neoadjuvant chemoradiotherapy is completed. If 45 Gy is used up front, as many still prefer, after the 1- to 2-month wait that occurs between clinical restaging and repeat lymph node biopsy if surgery is not provided and the patient is sent back for the completion of radiotherapy, the efficacy of the radiotherapy is dramatically diminished. For example, patients who have biopsy-proven recalcitrant (often called "persistent"), N2 disease have what is usually a contraindication for resection. The long gap that occurs during restaging and obtaining repeat biopsy to prove it makes the additional amount of radiation offered not as helpful as it would have been if it were given consecutively with the rest of the preoperative radiation.

For this reason we prefer to use doses of 60 Gy and, even more recently, 72 cGy in selected patients before resection. The main concern surgeons have is that surgery is not safe in this highly irradiated field, which is not true. A lobectomy can be performed safely in patients who have received high-dose preoperative radiation [13] if the bronchus is buttressed with a pedicled intercostal muscle flap that is harvested before placement of the chest retractor. We currently prefer to use an omental flap as the optimal bronchial buttressing for patients who undergo right pneumonectomy in a highly radiated field.

The ideal time to repeat a PET or PET/CT scan after radiotherapy or chemotherapy to best perform clinical restaging is currently unknown. In our experience, however, we find it to be accurate between 4 and 12 weeks [14,15]. In our practice, approximately 4 weeks after the completion of combined chemoradiotherapy, patients should be restaged by performing a repeat integrated PET/CT scan at the same center as the initial PET scan was performed. This step is critical because it allows for calculation of the change in the maxSUV values of the primary tumor and of the lymph nodes. This simple, easy-to-calculate value is a predictor of who has responded well to neoadjuvant therapy and who has not. Surgery, in general, should be reserved for patients who have been down-staged and have favorable biology.

Restaging, unlike initial staging, cannot always use mediastinal lymph node biopsy; however, repeat biopsies of the lymph nodes almost always should be tried. There exists one guiding principle about restaging: the mediastinal N2 lymph node that was proven to be positive before chemoradiotherapy should be re-biopsied after the completion of the neoadjuvant therapy using the same techniques used initially, unless it was mediastinoscopy. Although some researchers have shown that repeat mediastinoscopy is safe, in most surgical hands it is dangerous and inaccurate, especially after chest irradiation [16,17]. In 2002, Van Schil and associates [18] reported on 27 patients who underwent repeat mediastinoscopy after neoadjuvant therapy and found that 4 of the 16 (25%) patients had false-negative results. In 2000, Mateu-Navarro [16] reported on 24 patients, and 5 of the 12 had false-negative N2 disease results. We do not use repeat mediastinoscopy in our practice, although it is still the standard for some practices. Instead, we have used EBUS and EUS-FNA for our patients who had N2 disease diagnosed initially via mediastinoscopy. EUS-FNA is accurate for the 4R, 7, 8, and 9 stations for biopsy and re-biopsy; EBUS is good for stations 2R (if patients are not intubated during the procedure), 4R, 4L, and 7 locations. We use left VATS for sampling stations 5 and 6. Some surgeons have used EUS-FNA to re-biopsy stations 2R, 2L, 5, and 6, but few EUS endosonographers are unable to adequately visualize the lymph nodes in these stations. In 2003, Annema [19] reported 83% accuracy for repeat EUS-FNA in 19 patients after neoadjuvant chemoradiotherapy. If EBUS or EUS were used initially, then these same techniques should be repeated.

Often a surgeon is left with the clinical stage, as assessed via repeat PET/CT and CT, to guide him or her. We evaluated the accuracy of these repeat imaging modalities after neoadjuvant therapy. We performed several studies to evaluated the efficacy of restaging tests after chemoradiotherapy. The first study in 2003 [20] showed that repeat PET was more specific and had a higher positive predictive value and negative predictive value than repeat CT scan for detecting residual tumor in the lung in patients with NSCLC after neoadjuvant therapy. It also showed that repeat PET was more sensitive and more accurate for the restaging of the paratracheal (lymph node stations 2R and 4R) N2 lymph nodes. The change in the maxSUV continues to be an important and relatively new area of research. In our second study on restaging in 2004, we showed that the change in the maxSUV of the primary tumor on repeat PET held a near linear relationship with the pathologic response [21]. Our results may be secondary to the fact that we required the initial and repeat PET/CT to be performed on the same scanner with similar techniques. Ryu and colleagues [22] reported similar finding in 2002. Port and colleagues [23], however, concluded that repeat PET was not a good predictor of response. In that study, however, the authors did not mandate that the initial and repeat PET be performed at the same center. Therefore, this approach may afford better comparison.

In 2006, we first published a report stating that the maxSUV of mediastinal lymph nodes was a predictor of pathology, even in areas of the world that are endemic to histoplasmosis, a known common cause of false-positive results on PET scans [24]. In that study we found that when a maxSUV of 5.3 is used as a cut-off instead of the traditional 2.5, the accuracy for fluorodeoxyglucose (FDG)-PET-CT is increased to 92%. Even further, we showed that the ratio of the mediastinal lymph node to the primary tumor may be the best predictor of pathology and may take into account the different techniques used by different PET centers [25]. First we showed that maxSUV of lymph nodes and the primary tumor predicts pathology before chemoradiotherapy. Then in a study published in 2006 [15] we revealed that the accuracy of repeat PET/CT was best for complete responders (92%) and for patients with stage I disease (89%); however, it fell to only 69% for patients with persistent stage III disease. From this study we also showed that the change in the maxSUV after neoadjuvant chemoradiotherapy was predictive of response. Most importantly from our restaging paper we found that the percentage of change and not the absolute value of the repeat PET/CT is predictive. When the maxSUV of the primary tumor decreases by 75% or more, it is highly likely (+LR, 6.1) that the patient is a complete responder. When it decreases by 55% or more, it is highly likely (+LR, 9.1) that the patient is a partial responder. When the mass of the N2 nodes initially involved with metastatic cancer decreases by more than 50% it is highly likely (+LR, 7.9) that the node is rendered benign. The change in the maxSUV of the primary tumor is predictive and the change in the maxSUV of lymph nodes that were initially biopsy proven is predicative of pathology.

This finding represents a powerful way to guide one's practice. For example, if the maxSUV of a 4R lymph node was 12, mediastinoscopy proved it was positive and only N2 disease, and after neoadjuvant therapy the repeat maxSUV 1 month later was node 3, this is a reliable sign of response. A negative result on EBUS of that node indicates immediately advancement to thoracotomy and resection in our practice. If the maxSUV was 10 on the repeat PET/CT and the EBUS was negative, however, we may start off with a VATS instead of a thoracotomy and try to biopsy the node and send it for frozen section. The decrease in size of the lymph node on repeat CT scan is not a reliable way to determine the pathologic change in a node. If the node is much smaller, it is often helpful; if it is larger or the same size, then little information is yielded.

In conclusion, restaging patients with NSCLC who had stage IIIA cancer from N2 disease is valuable. It help guides the type of preoperative therapy given and the selective use of surgery after its completion. Because survival after resection is poor for patients with recalcitrant N2 disease, surgical resection generally should be offered only exclusively to patients who have been down-staged and are rendered N2 negative. The repeat staging should be as thorough as the initial staging. Tissue biopsies must be performed initially to ensure that a patient is stage IIIA and not less or more. Then repeat staging can stand on the shoulders of the initial PET. If the maxSUV of a lymph node falls and it was previously negative, it does not need to be rebiopsied. If the maxSUV rises, however, then that node may require biopsy. If lymph nodes or M1 sites were not initially biopsied and assumptions were made, then the repeat staging is less interpretable because the patient's initial stage was never determined accurately. If the initial stage was accurate, we prefer to re-biopsy lymph nodes that were proven to be malignant. We prefer the use of EBUS or EUS-FNA. We do not use repeat mediastinoscopy. Finally, the percent change in the maxSUV of the mediastinal nodes and the primary tumor is the most accurate clinical predictor of biologic response rate. It should be calculated and carefully considered to help guide clinical decisions and select procedures for biopsy of specific targets.

References

[1] National Cancer Institute. Surveillance, epidemiology and end results (SEER) public use data 1973–2002. Available at: http://seer.cancer.gov/publicdata. Accessed June 15, 2005.

[2] Cerfolio RJ, Bryant AS. Survival of patients with unsuspected N2 (stage IIIA) non small-cell lung cancer. Ann Thorac Surg 2008;86:362–6.

[3] Cerfolio RJ, Maniscalco LM, Bryant AS. The treatment of patients with stage IIIA non-small cell lung cancer from N2 disease: who returns to the surgical arena and who survives? Ann Thorac Surg 2008; 86:912–20.

[4] Rosell R, Gomez-Codina J, Camps C, et al. Preresectional chemotherapy in stage IIIA non-small-cell lung cancer: a 7-year assessment of a randomized controlled trial. Lung Cancer 1999;26:7–14.

[5] Roth J, Fossella F, Komaki R, et al. A randomized trial comparing perioperative chemotherapy and surgery with surgery alone in resectable stage IIIA non-small-cell lung cancer. J Natl Cancer Inst 1994;86:673–80.

[6] Detterbeck F, Socinski M. Induction chemotherapy and surgery for I-III A, B non-small cell lung cancer. In: Detterbeck F, Socinski M, Rivera M, et al, editors. Diagnosis and treatment of lung cancer: an evidence-based guide for the practicing clinician. Philadelphia: WB Saunders Co; 2001. p. 267–82.

[7] Bueno R, Richards W, Swanson S, et al. Nodal stage after induction therapy for stage IIIA lung cancer determines patient survival. Ann Thorac Surg 2000;70:1826–31.

[8] Voltolini L, Luzzi L, Ghiribelli C, et al. Results of induction chemotherapy followed by surgical resection in patients with stage IIIA (N2) non-small cell lung cancer the importance of the nodal down-staging after chemotherapy. Eur J Cardiothorac Surg 2001; 20:1106–12.

[9] Komaki R, Cox JD, Hartz AJ, et al. Characteristics of long-term survivors after treatment for inoperable carcinoma of the lung. Am J Clin Oncol 1985;8:362–70.

[10] Cerfolio RJ, Bryant AS, Eloubeidi MA. Routine mediastinoscopy and esophageal ultrasound fine-needle aspiration in patients with non-small cell lung cancer who are clinically N2 negative: a prospective study. Chest 2006;130:1791–5.

[11] Smith MA, Battafarno RJ, Meyers RF, et al. Prevalence of benign disease in patients undergoing

resection for suspected lung cancer. Ann Thorac Surg 2006;81:1824–8.

[12] Cerfolio RJ, Bryant AS, Spencer SA, et al. Pulmonary resection after high-dose and low-dose chest irradiation. Ann Thorac Surg 2005;80:1224–30.

[13] Cerfolio RJ, Bryant AS, Yamamuro M. Intercostal muscle flap to buttress the bronchus at risk and the thoracic esophageal-gastric anastamosis. Ann Thorac Surg 2005;80:1017–20.

[14] Cerfolio RJ, Bryant AS. When is it best to repeat a 2-fluoro-2-deoxy-D-glucose positron emission tomography/computed tomography scan on patients with non-small cell lung cancer who have received neoadjuvant chemoradiotherapy? Ann Thorac Surg 2007; 84:1092–7.

[15] Cerfolio RJ, Bryant AS, Ojha B. Restaging patients with N2 (stage IIIa) non-small cell lung cancer after neoadjuvant chemoradiotherapy: a prospective study. J Thorac Cardiovasc Surg 2006;131:1229–35.

[16] Mateu-Navarro M, Rami-Porta R, Bastus-Piulats R, et al. Remediastinoscopy after induction chemotherapy in non-small cell lung cancer. Ann Thorac Surg 2000;70:391–5.

[17] Pitz C, Mass K, Swieten H, et al. Surgery as part of combined modality treatment in stage IIIB non-small cell lung cancer. Ann Thorac Surg 2002;74: 164–9.

[18] Van Schil P, Schoot van der J, Poniewierski J, et al. Remediastinoscopy after neoadjuvant therapy for non-small cell lung cancer. Lung Cancer 2002;37: 281–5.

[19] Annema JT, Veselic M, Versteegh MI, et al. Mediastinal restaging: EUS-FNA offers a new perspective. Lung Cancer 2003;42:311–8.

[20] Cerfolio RJ, Ojha B, Mukherjee S, et al. Positron emission tomography scanning with 2-fluoro-2-deoxyglucose as a predictor of response for non-small cell cancer. J Thorac Cardiovasc Surg 2003; 125:938–44.

[21] Cerfolio RJ, Bryant AS, Winokur TS, et al. Repeat FDG-PET after neoadjuvant therapy is a predictor of pathologic response in patients with non-small cell lung cancer. Ann Thorac Surg 2004;78:1903–9.

[22] Ryu JS, Choi NC, Fischman AJ, et al. FDG-PET in staging and restaging non-small cell lung cancer after neoadjuvant chemoradiotherapy: correlation with histopathology. Lung Cancer 2002;35:179–87.

[23] Port JL, Kent MS, Korst RJ, et al. Positron emission tomography scanning poorly predicts response to preoperative chemotherapy in non-small cell lung cancer. Ann Thorac Surg 2004;77:254–9.

[24] Bryant AS, Cerfolio RJ, Klemm KM, et al. Maximum standard uptake value of mediastinal lymph nodes on integrated FDG-PET-CT predicts pathology in patients with non-small cell lung cancer. Ann Thorac Surg 2006;82:417–22.

[25] Cerfolio RJ, Bryant AS. Ratio of the maximum standardized uptake value on FDG-PET of the mediastinal (N2) lymph node to the primary tumor may be a universal predictor of nodal malignancy in patients with non-small cell lung cancer. Ann Thorac Surg 2007;83:1826–30.

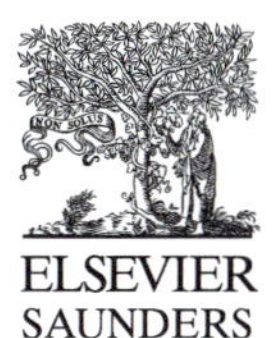

ELSEVIER
SAUNDERS

Thorac Surg Clin 18 (2008) 423–435

THORACIC
SURGERY
CLINICS

Adjuvant Therapy for Non–Small Cell Lung Cancer with Mediastinal Nodal Involvement

Rachel E. Sanborn, MD[a,*], Brian E. Lally, MD[b]

[a]Providence Portland Medical Center, 4805 NE Glisan Street, 2N35, Portland, OR 97213, USA

[b]Fox Chase Cancer Center, Department of Radiation Oncology, 333 Cottman Avenue, Philadelphia, PA 19111, USA

Lung cancer is the most common cause of cancer-related mortality in the United States and worldwide [1,2]. Non–small-cell lung cancer (NSCLC) represents most cases of lung cancers. Most patients are unfortunately diagnosed at an advanced and incurable stage [3]. Even in patients with clinically diagnosed early-stage disease, occult mediastinal nodal metastases may be found in 3% to 21% of patients at the time of resection [4]. The presence of ipsilateral mediastinal lymph node involvement (N2 disease) is a marker of poor prognosis, with 5-year survival rates with resection alone of 3% to 34% [5,6]. Poor survival is caused by the increased likelihood of undetected micrometastatic disease before surgical resection. The poor outcomes of this population subset in NSCLC have led to ongoing efforts to improve presurgical staging and improve upon survival with combined modality therapies.

For patients with established mediastinal lymph node involvement, the role and timing of treatment with different modalities (eg, chemotherapy, radiotherapy, or surgery) are controversial. In patients with bulky mediastinal disease, any role at all for surgical resection is questionable [7]. This article focuses on adjuvant treatment options for resected NSCLC with N2 involvement. The evidence for and roles of neoadjuvant therapy for N2 disease in NSCLC and definitive chemoradiotherapy for locally advanced NSCLC are addressed in other articles in this issue.

Difficulties of mediastinal staging

Evaluation of the mediastinum for disease involvement with NSCLC may be accomplished in various ways. Clinical staging may be performed with CT. CT scanning of the chest is useful in providing anatomic detail, but the accuracy of chest CT scanning in differentiating benign from malignant lymph nodes in the mediastinum is poor. The accuracy of CT is inferior when compared to the accuracy of staging with positron emission tomography (PET) [8]. In a prospective evaluation of 102 patients with NSCLC, clinical staging with CT demonstrated 75% sensitivity and 66% specificity for the detection of mediastinal metastases. The corresponding values for staging PET were 91% and 86%, with PET results significantly correlating with the pathologic results of surgical mediastinal lymph node evaluation ($P < .001$). When evaluated for the detection of mediastinal nodal involvement and distant metastases, PET demonstrated 95% sensitivity and 83% specificity [8]. Despite the improvement in detection, clinical staging can be hampered by false-positive and false-negative results, including with the use of integrated PET/CT [9–11]. PET scanning has much better sensitivity and specificity than chest CT scanning for staging lung cancer in the mediastinum, and distant metastatic disease can be detected by PET scanning. With either test, abnormal findings must be confirmed by tissue biopsy to ensure accurate staging [12].

Pathologic evaluation of the mediastinum offers the advantage of potentially more accurate identification of lymph node involvement; however, the

* Corresponding author.
E-mail address: rachel.sanborn@providence.org (R.E. Sanborn).

doi:10.1016/j.thorsurg.2008.08.004

approaches are necessarily more invasive. Mediastinoscopy and video-assisted thoracoscopy are the most common approaches for surgical evaluation of the mediastinum. Each approach offers limitations regarding accessibility of lymph nodes and requiring an invasive procedure. Less invasive approaches with endoscopic or endobronchial ultrasonography offer attractive alternatives to the above procedures. In a small randomized trial (40 patients) of patients with NSCLC that required mediastinal evaluation, endoscopic ultrasonography demonstrated 93% sensitivity compared to 73% sensitivity with surgical staging (mediastinoscopy in 20 patients and anterior mediastinotomy in 1 patient) [13].

Endoscopic ultrasonography and endobronchial ultrasonography were evaluated in combination with transbronchial needle aspiration in a series of 138 patients undergoing mediastinal staging as part of an evaluation for suspected lung cancer [14]. Endobronchial ultrasonography was more sensitive than transbronchial needle aspiration in detecting malignant lymph node involvement (69% versus 36%, $P = .003$). Endoscopic ultrasonography and endobronchial ultrasonography in combination demonstrated a higher estimated sensitivity and negative predictive value (93% and 97%, respectively) than did either method alone (sensitivities 69% each alone and negative predictive values 88% each alone; *P* value not reported) [14].

The field of mediastinal staging is evolving. Currently, mediastinoscopy is still regarded as the gold standard before surgical resection. Despite improvements in techniques, all staging approaches may fail to identify small-volume mediastinal lymph node metastases, which may be identified subsequently on the final pathologic specimen after a complete surgical resection. Physicians then must evaluate which adjuvant therapeutic approaches may offer patients the greatest survival benefit.

Adjuvant chemotherapy

Before the development of cisplatin, the addition of chemotherapy after surgical resection did not provide a survival benefit and unfortunately showed evidence of causing harm [15]. The publication of a meta-analysis in 1995, which included 4357 patients with resected NSCLC, provided the first indications of improvement in survival compared to surgical resection alone for patients treated with cisplatin-based therapies. Although the results were not statistically significant, findings indicated a 5% benefit in survival at 5 years with cisplatin-based adjuvant chemotherapy [15].

This meta-analysis prompted a randomized trial of adjuvant chemotherapy versus observation for patients undergoing resection of NSCLC (International Adjuvant Lung Trial [IALT]). Patients undergoing complete resection of stages I through III NSCLC were randomized to receive three or four cycles of cisplatin-based adjuvant chemotherapy versus observation. The trial allowed for postoperative radiation to be administered at the discretion of the participating institutions. Of the 1867 patients enrolled, 734 had stage III disease, with 479 patients having pathologic N2 disease. Overall, the trial confirmed an absolute 5-year survival benefit of 4.1% for patients undergoing adjuvant chemotherapy ($P < .03$), with subset analysis confirming a survival benefit in patients with stage III disease [16]. In subsequent long-term follow up at 7.5 years, the investigators reported a loss in the overall- and disease-free survival benefits in comparison to the planned 5-year analysis (hazard ratio for overall survival 0.86 at 5 years and 1.45 beyond 5 years, *P* value for interaction 0.006; hazard ratio for disease-free survival 0.85 at 5 years and 1.33 beyond 5 years, *P* value for interaction 0.04). Although this trial was not powered for the long-term follow-up, the investigators raised the concern for possible chemotherapy-related "over mortality" in the long-term and the need for long-term follow-up in clinical trials [17].

In another phase III randomized trial (Adjuvant Navelbine International Trialist Association [ANITA]), 840 patients with resected stage IB-IIIA NSCLC were administered four cycles of adjuvant cisplatin in combination with vinorelbine. Three hundred twenty-five patients (39%) had stage IIIA disease, with 224 patients having N2 involvement. The ANITA trial confirmed a benefit in survival with adjuvant chemotherapy, with the median survival 65.7 months with chemotherapy compared with 43.7 months for controls, and a hazard ratio 0.8 for chemotherapy compared to controls ($P = .017$). The absolute 5-year survival benefit was 8.6% with chemotherapy, with the survival benefit persisting at 8.4% at 7 years [18].

A subgroup analysis of the ANITA trial indicated a nonsignificant trend toward increased survival benefit in more advanced compared with earlier-stage disease (5-year survival of stages IB: 62% chemo versus 64% control; stage II: 52% versus 39%; and stage IIIA: 42% versus 26%, respectively; $P = .07$). Subgroup analysis according to lymph node station involvement indicated a nonsignificant trend toward increasing survival benefit in patients with more advanced lymph node station involvement (5-year survival of N0 status: 58% chemo versus 61% control; N1 status: 52% versus 36%; N2 status: 40% versus 19%, respectively) [18]. The authors concluded that because of the low number of patients in each subgroup, definitive conclusions could not be drawn based on the results of this study alone [18].

Cisplatin-based chemotherapy combinations have not been universally shown to have equal outcomes and survival benefits. The Adjuvant Lung Project of Italy (ALPI) was a randomized phase III trial involving 1209 patients with resected stages I-IIIA NSCLC [19]. Patients were randomized to receive three cycles of cisplatin with mitomycin and vindesine (MVP) versus observation alone. Three hundred ten patients enrolled in the trial had stage IIIA disease, with 272 patients having N2 involvement. Because of concerns regarding data integrity, only 1088 patients were analyzed for survival. The hazard ratio for survival was 0.96 for chemotherapy versus controls ($P = .589$), indicating there was no benefit with the administration of MVP chemotherapy after surgical resection of NSCLC. Subset analysis failed to identify an interaction between treatment and disease stage for improvement in outcome, although the study did confirm shorter overall- and progression-free survival with more advanced-stage disease in either arm [19].

The reasons for the negative outcome of the ALPI trial are not certain. The MVP regimen was associated with poor compliance (22% of patients stopped treatment early because of toxicity) and a high incidence of early death (90 patients in the MVP arm and 69 patients in the control arm) [19]. It may be that the toxicity of the selected regimen was such that patients received an inadequate total chemotherapy dose.

In the Big Lung Trial, 381 patients with resectable lung cancer were randomized to receive three cycles of cisplatin-based therapy versus no chemotherapy [20]. Patients were not enrolled by specific tumor stage, but rather by the criteria of surgery being the "treatment of choice." Chemotherapy could be administered either before or after surgical resection, although only 3% of patients received neoadjuvant chemotherapy (compared with 97% receiving adjuvant chemotherapy). The study failed to identify a survival benefit for patients receiving chemotherapy compared with observation (median survival 33.9 months with chemotherapy versus 32.6 months without chemotherapy). The hazard ratio in favor of no chemotherapy was 1.02 ($P = .90$) [20]. There was no evidence in subgroup analysis for differential survival outcomes among different disease stages, including the 99 patients with stage IIIA disease. The study acknowledged that it was not statistically powered to detect a survival benefit, even if the goal enrollment of 500 patients had been met [20]. The lack of statistical power with small sample size prevents conclusions regarding a possible benefit of chemotherapy.

The Lung Adjuvant Cisplatin Evaluation analysis was a pooled analysis of five randomized trials of adjuvant chemotherapy. This meta-analysis included updated patient information of 4584 patients enrolled into randomized trials of adjuvant chemotherapy for resected NSCLC [21]. Twenty-seven percent of patients had stage III disease. With a median follow-up of 5 years, the hazard ratio for survival was 0.84, favoring adjuvant chemotherapy as opposed to controls ($P < .001$). This translated into a 5.5% absolute survival benefit at 5 years. In subgroup analysis, the hazard ratio for stage III disease was 0.83 (P value not reported) [21]. The meta-analysis did not report on survival separated by nodal status.

Uracil-tegafur (UFT) is an orally available chemotherapeutic agent that acts as a precursor to 5-fluorouracil. The agent has been studied in the adjuvant setting for NSCLC primarily in the Japanese population. In the setting of resected stage I-III NSCLC, Imaizumi and colleagues [22] evaluated 309 patients randomized to receive one cycle of cisplatin with adriamycin, followed by 6 months of UFT, versus observation alone. Although 43 patients in the treatment arm and 35 patients in the control arm had stage III disease, only 27 patients in the treatment arm and 20 patients in the control arm had N2 disease. The two arms of the study had not been stratified for prognostic factors, and N2 status differed significantly in the trial. On initial evaluation, no difference was detected in survival, with 5-year survival of 61.8% in the treatment arm versus 58.1% in the control arm ($P = .223$). After adjustment for N stage, a significant survival benefit with adjuvant chemotherapy was detected, although the exact survival rates were not reported [22]. The authors concluded that after adjustment for nodal status, adjuvant chemotherapy demonstrated a survival benefit. The lack of reporting of the specific benefit and the lack of prospective stratification hampered definitive conclusions from this trial.

In a large three-arm randomized phase III trial, Wada and colleagues [23] evaluated UFT in patients with resected stage I-IIIA NSCLC. Patients were randomized to receive cisplatin and vindesine for three cycles followed by 1-year administration of UFT, UFT alone for 1 year, or surgery alone. Of the 310 patients randomized and eligible for evaluation, 42 had pathologic N2 involvement, and 55 patients had stage IIIA disease. The 5-year survival rate for cisplatin-based chemotherapy with UFT was 60.6% and with UFT alone was 64.1%, compared with the control arm of 49%. The administration of adjuvant chemotherapy demonstrated survival benefit when compared to surgery alone ($P = .044$), with UFT alone demonstrating the most favorable comparison (hazard ratio 0.55; $P = .022$) [23].

Nakagawa and associates [24] evaluated 267 patients with resected stage I-IIIA NSCLC in a phase III randomized trial. Patients with resected stage II or IIIA disease were randomized to receive two cycles of cisplatin with vindesine followed by 1 year of UFT or observation alone. N2 disease was noted in 51 patients enrolled in the trial, with 62 patients having stage IIIA disease. Although significant survival benefits were detected for patients with stage I disease receiving adjuvant chemotherapy, no difference in survival was seen for patients with more advanced disease (8-year overall survival rate was 36.8% for controls versus 38% with chemotherapy; $P = .52$) [24].

In a phase III trial that specifically involved patients with resected stage IIIA-N2 NSCLC, Tanaka and colleagues [25] randomized 58 patients to receive either one or two cycles of cisplatin and vindesine followed by 1 year of UFT or UFT for 1 year alone. No differences were detected in the 5-year overall survival rate (46% and 47%, respectively; $P = .401$) [25]. The small number of patients enrolled in this phase III trial and the lack of a control arm make determinations regarding the relative benefit of UFT difficult.

A meta-analysis of adjuvant UFT in resected NSCLC was conducted that involved updated patient information from six randomized controlled trials [26]. Most of the 2003 patients had stage I disease (number of patients with N2 disease not reported). Treatment with adjuvant UFT was associated with improved 5-year and 7-year overall survival rates (81.5% and 76.5%, respectively) compared with surgery alone (77.2% and 69.5%; $P = .011$ and .001, respectively) [26]. Multivariate analysis indicated a benefit after adjustment for nodal status (N0 versus N1-3), with a hazard ratio for adjuvant therapy of 0.75 ($P = .002$) [26].

The largest meta-analysis of adjuvant chemotherapy incorporated updated patient information involving 8147 patients enrolled in 30 randomized controlled trials [27]. Cisplatin-based chemotherapy without UFT was administered in 15 of the trials, whereas 7 trials administered UFT with cisplatin and 8 trials evaluated UFT alone. Seventeen percent of patients had stage IIIA disease at resection. The pooled analysis of all clinical trials yielded a highly significant hazard ratio of 0.87 favoring adjuvant chemotherapy ($P < .000001$), which translated into an absolute benefit in survival at 5 years of 4% (60% 5-year survival rate for controls versus 64% rate with chemotherapy) and an absolute benefit in survival rate at 8 years of 5%. The meta-analysis was unable to identify a clear indication of a difference in effect between different chemotherapeutic regimens or between disease stage and differences in survival benefit [27].

At this time the use of UFT remains limited to Japanese populations, as the agent has not been tested in other populations. Preferential administration of UFT is in patients with earlier stage disease, in whom the bulk of the data regarding survival benefit lies. Conclusions regarding any benefit in more advanced disease and in non-Asian populations cannot be made. The bulk of evidence supporting a survival benefit in resected NSCLC, including stage IIIA disease, is with the administration of cisplatin-based chemotherapy. Although the Lung Adjuvant Cisplatin Evaluation meta-analysis noted superior survival with the combination of cisplatin with vinorelbine (hazard ratio 0.80, $P = .04$) compared to other cisplatin-based combinations, it was recognized that the patients administered vinorelbine received a higher total dose of cisplatin [21]. The authors concluded that the relative survival benefit may relate to the higher dose of cisplatin as opposed to the vinorelbine itself [21].

Table 1 lists the trials of adjuvant chemotherapy, including patients with stage IIIA NSCLC. Table 2 lists the meta-analyses of adjuvant chemotherapy involving patients with stage IIIA NSCLC.

Adjuvant radiotherapy

The role of adjuvant radiation in the treatment of resected NSCLC is controversial. The

Table 1
Phase III trials of adjuvant chemotherapy including stage IIIA non–small-cell lung cancer

Trial	Disease stage	Chemotherapy regimen	Number of patients	Number with N2	Survival	*P* value
IALT [16]	I-III	Cisplatin-based × 4 cycles vs Obs	1867	479	4.1% Absolute 5-y surv benefit	$P < .03$
ANITA [18]	IB-IIIA	Cisplatin/vinorelbine × 4 cycles vs Obs	840	224	Med surv: 65.7 mo vs 43.7 mo; HR = 0.08; 5-y surv benefit: 8.6%	$P = .017$
ALPI [19]	I-IIIA	Cisplatin, mitomycin, vindesine × 3 cycles vs Obs	1088	272	HR = 0.96	$P = .589$
Big Lung Trial [20]	"Resectable"	Cisplatin-based × 3 cycles vs Obs	381	99 (IIIA)	Med surv: 33.9 mo vs 32.6 mo HR = 1.02	$P = .90$
Imaizumi et al [22]	I-III	Cisplatin/adriamycin × 1 cycle, then UFT × 6 mo vs Obs	309	47	5-y surv: 61.8% vs 58.1%	$P = .223$
Wada et al [23]	I-IIIA	Cisplatin/vindesine × 3 cycles, then UFT × 12 mo; vs UFT × 12 mo; vs Obs	310	42	5-y surv: 60.6% with chemo/UFT; 64.1% UFT; 49% Obs HR with UFT vs Obs: 0.55	$P = .044$ (Chemo/UFT vs Obs) $P = .022$ (HR UFT vs Obs)
Nagakawa et al [24]	I-IIIA	Cisplatin/vindesine × 2 cycles, then UFT × 12 mo; vs Obs	267	51	8-y OS: 38% vs 36.8%	$P = .52$
Tanaka et al [25]	IIIA (N2)	Cisplatin/vindesine × 1 or 2 cycles, then UFT × 12 mo; vs UFT × 12 mo	58	58	5-y OS: 46% vs 47%	$P = .401$

Abbreviations: 5-y surv, 5-year survival; HR, hazard ratio; Med surv, median survival; Mo, months; NR, not reported; Obs, observation; UFT, uracil-tegafur.

Table 2
Meta-analyses of adjuvant chemotherapy involving stage IIIA non—small-cell lung cancer

Trial	Disease stage	Chemotherapy regimen	Number of patients	Overall survival	*P* value
Brit Med Journal [15]	I-IV	Numerous	9387 total;1394 pts with resected NSCLC with cisplatin-based therapy	HR: 0.87 Abs 5-y surv benefit: 5%	*P* = .08
LACE [21]	Resected I-III	Cisplatin-based	4584	HR: 0.84 5-y surv benefit: 5.5%	*P* <.001
Hamada et al [26]	Resected	UFT vs Obs	2003	5-y surv: 81.5% vs 77.2% 7-y surv: 76.5% vs 69.5%	*P* = .011 *P* = .001
Stewart et al [27]	I-IIIB	Cisplatin-based; cisplatin-based with UFT; UFT alone	8147	HR 0.86 Abs 5-y surv benefit 4%	*P* <.000001

Abbreviations: Abs 5-y surv, absolute 5-year survival; HR, hazard ratio; NSCLC, non–small-cell lung cancer; Obs, observation; Pts, patients; UFT, uracil-tegafur.

postoperative radiotherapy (PORT) meta-analysis evaluated updated information from 2128 patients from nine randomized clinical trials [28]. The meta-analysis demonstrated an overall detriment in survival with the administration of adjuvant radiation for resected NSCLC, with a hazard ratio of 1.21 ($P = .001$) and a 21% increase in the relative risk of death with adjuvant radiation compared to controls. This corresponded to an absolute detriment in 2-year survival rate of 7%, reducing 2-year survival rates overall from 55% to 48% [28]. Subgroup analyses were conducted evaluating survival by disease stage and nodal status. The detriment of PORT was inversely related to nodal status, with significantly reduced survival noted for N0 and N1 disease. The results for stage III and N2 patients favored PORT, although the difference was not significant. The authors concluded that there was no clear evidence of an adverse effect for patients with stage III, N2, resected NSCLC administered adjuvant radiation and that further research in this disease stage was warranted [28].

Updated information of the PORT meta-analysis included one further trial with the addition of 104 patients, with a total of 2232 patients evaluated [29]. The updated analysis reached similar conclusions, noting an 18% increase in the relative risk of death with PORT overall ($P = .002$), with an absolute detriment in 2-year survival rate of 6%. Overall survival rate decreased from 58% without PORT to 52% with PORT. Again, no clear evidence of detriment to survival was detected in the subset analysis of N2 disease [29].

Several concerns have been raised regarding the 1998 PORT meta-analysis [30–33]. Trials that were included in the meta-analysis used radiation techniques that currently are recognized as less than optimal, particularly lateral radiation beam designs and relatively large radiation fields [34]. Treatment with cobalt-60 teletherapy units was allowed in seven of the nine trials, and four trials used relatively large daily radiation fractionation schedules (> 2 Gy/day); both of these techniques have been associated with increased normal tissue toxicity [35,36]. Taken together, these critical components of radiation delivery may have deleterious consequences in a population of patients with already compromised cardiac and pulmonary reserve. Given these "faults" of the analysis, a retrospective analysis of the Surveillance, Epidemiology, and End Results (SEER) database was conducted, which evaluated patients who had resected stage II or III NSCLC administered adjuvant radiotherapy or were undergoing observation during a time in which the linear accelerator was standard for radiation delivery [37]. The analysis included 7465 patients, with 47% receiving PORT. Overall, PORT was not shown to impact survival (hazard ratio 1.048, $P = .1269$). Subset analysis by nodal status confirmed the findings of the PORT meta-analysis, demonstrating a significant decrease in survival for patients with N0 or N1 disease administered PORT (hazard ratio 1.1176 and 1.097; $P = .0435$ and .0196, respectively). For patients with N2 disease, however, a significant benefit in survival was noted with the addition of PORT (hazard ratio 0.855, $P = .0077$) [37].

An additional study involving the SEER database was designed to investigate whether the mortality from heart disease, a manifestation of intercurrent disease after PORT, has decreased over time for patients with NSCLC. The results from this study demonstrated that the risk of heart disease mortality associated with PORT has declined in more recent years, which may be secondary to improvements in the treatment planning and delivery of thoracic radiotherapy [38]. A descriptive analysis of PORT outcomes within the ANITA study noted an apparent improvement in overall survival for patients with N2 disease, regardless of chemotherapy administration (no statistical evaluation reported). The 5-year overall survival rate for N2 disease receiving PORT was 47% for patients treated with adjuvant chemotherapy and 21% for patients receiving PORT on the observation arm. This rate compares to a 34% 5-year survival rate with adjuvant chemotherapy and no PORT and 17% for the observation arm without PORT [18]. The more promising results of these more modern series have supported the rationale for ongoing prospective study of PORT in resected N2 NSCLC.

Currently a multi-institutional phase III trial is ongoing in Europe. It randomizes patients with resected NSCLC with N2 disease, regardless of chemotherapy administration, to receive three-dimensional conformal PORT versus no PORT [39]. The primary endpoint of the Lung Adjuvant Radiotherapy Trial is to detect a 10% difference in 3-year disease-free survival. Seven hundred patients are required [39].

Outside of a clinical trial, current guidelines from the American Society of Clinical Oncology and Cancer Care Ontario and the American College of Chest Physicians state that adjuvant radiation is not recommended for routine use for resected stage IIIA NSCLC because of the "lack of prospective randomized clinical trial data evaluating its efficacy" [40,41].

Adjuvant chemoradiotherapy

The combination of concurrent chemotherapy and radiation has been evaluated with mixed results. In the largest randomized trial, the Eastern Cooperative Oncology Group randomized 488 patients with resected lung cancer to receive adjuvant cisplatin and etoposide concurrently with radiation versus adjuvant radiation alone (ECOG 3590 trial) [42]. One hundred thirty-six patients (out of 246 patients total) in the chemoradiation arm had N2 disease, compared with 129 patients in the radiation control arm (out of 242 total patients). Median survival for the entire group was 38 months in the chemoradiation arm and 39 months in the control arm ($P = .56$). When survival was evaluated by disease stage (separated by stage II versus IIIA, not by nodal status), no difference in survival was detected. Toxicity was greater in the chemoradiation arm, with four deaths caused by sepsis, pneumonitis, and esophagitis. Two deaths from radiation-induced pneumonitis and one from esophagitis also occurred in the control arm. The authors concluded from this study that adjuvant chemoradiation did not have any clear benefit over radiation alone and that further study should be restricted to clinical trials [42].

The Radiation Therapy Oncology Group conducted a nonrandomized phase II study of concurrent carboplatin and paclitaxel administered with radiation for patients with resected stage II and IIIA NSCLC (RTOG 9705 study) [43]. Of 88 patients eligible for evaluation, 42 had N2 disease. The median survival for patients in this phase II study was 56.3 months, which the authors noted compared favorably with the previously mentioned study. The authors acknowledged that cross-comparison of survival between a nonrandomized phase II study and a randomized phase III trial is not recommended but concluded that further evaluation in clinical trials was warranted [43].

In a nonrandomized phase II feasibility study, Greco and colleagues [44] administered three cycles of adjuvant carboplatin and paclitaxel followed by concurrent carboplatin, paclitaxel, and thoracic radiation to 67 patients with resected stages II to IV (ipsilateral lung nodules) NSCLC. Thirty-three of 84 patients eligible in this series had resected N2 disease. With a short follow-up, 65% of patients were progression-free at 10 months. Grade 3 or 4 esophagitis occurred in 27% of patients treated with chemoradiation, and 11 patients required hospitalization for severe esophagitis. Radiation-induced pneumonitis was noted in 2% of patients treated, with 1 patient requiring hospitalization. The authors concluded that the regimen was feasible and well tolerated overall and that further evaluation in phase III trials was warranted for stage III resected NSCLC [44].

Currently, given the lack of phase III evidence demonstrating survival benefit, concurrent chemoradiation in the adjuvant setting is recommended only within the context of a clinical trial.

Prophylactic cranial irradiation

Despite the survival benefits of adjuvant systemic therapy, distant relapse after resection of locally advanced NSCLC frequently occurs. Relapses in the brain have been noted in 30% to 53% of patients with resected stage IIIA (N2) NSCLC [45,46]. Despite the proven survival benefit of prophylactic cranial irradiation (PCI) in limited stage small-cell lung cancer and extensive stage small-cell lung cancer [47,48], evidence regarding a survival benefit in NSCLC is lacking. Recent efforts to conduct a randomized phase III trial of PCI versus observation after completion of definitive therapy for locally advanced NSCLC (RTOG 0214), with the primary goal of evaluating possible survival benefit, closed because of poor accrual [49].

Pottgen and colleagues [50] conducted a randomized trial in patients who had surgically resectable locally advanced NSCLC. Treatment in the control arm involved surgical resection followed by adjuvant thoracic radiation therapy to 50 Gy. Patients enrolled in the experimental arm received neoadjuvant chemotherapy with three cycles of cisplatin and etoposide, followed by chemoradiation (to a total of 45 Gy) with cisplatin and etoposide and definitive surgery. Patients in the chemotherapy arm received PCI. The trial was hampered by use of the older lung cancer staging criteria and slow accrual, which necessitated trial closure before completion of accrual. Pathologic nodal involvement was not reported. For the 106 patients eligible for evaluation, 5-year overall survival rate was 18% in the control arm versus 16% in the chemotherapy and PCI arm ($P = .15$). Brain relapse occurred in 9 patients in the control arm and 4 patients in the PCI arm. When comparing patients who received PCI to those who did not, the 5-year probability of brain relapse was 7.8% for patients receiving PCI versus 34.7% for patients who did not ($P = .01$). The authors concluded that PCI significantly reduced the rate brain metastases and acknowledged the small number of patients enrolled in their study for which PCI outcomes were not the primary endpoint [50].

Given the paucity of data at this time, the routine use of PCI is not recommended outside of a clinical trial. Poor accrual to clinical studies to evaluate this question, however, has currently placed a frustrating halt to ongoing investigation without a definitive answer.

Treatment in the elderly population

Despite the increasing proportion of patients over the age of 70 diagnosed with lung cancer in the United States, elderly patients continue to be underrepresented in clinical trials. Dedicated analyses of adjuvant chemotherapy in elderly patients with resected NSCLC are limited, and analyses of elderly patients treated with adjuvant therapy for resected locally advanced NSCLC do not exist.

The National Cancer Institute of Canada Clinical Trials Group evaluated outcomes of elderly patients enrolled in their study of adjuvant cisplatin and vinorelbine versus observation for resected stage IB or stage II NSCLC (the JBR.10 study) [51]. Elderly patients were defined in this analysis as persons over the age of 65. Of 482 patients enrolled in the trial, 155 were defined as elderly, with 77 patients in the chemotherapy arm and 78 patients in the observation arm. Subset analyses were conducted to stratify patients by age groups of 65 years and younger, 66 to 70 years old, 71 to 75 years, and over 75 years (327, 84, 48, and 23 patients, respectively). Despite the fact that elderly patients had a poorer baseline performance status and received less chemotherapy than younger patients, adjuvant cisplatin-based chemotherapy resulted in an overall survival benefit in the elderly population similar to the results of the overall trial population (hazard ratio 0.61; $P = .04$). In subset analyses, the stratified age ranges experienced overall survival benefits, with the exception of patients over the age of 75 (hazard ratio 2.41; $P < .001$ compared to younger patients). This subset analysis was limited by the fact that it only contained 12 patients in the chemotherapy arm and 11 patients in the observation arm. It was noted that in this subset, the same benefit in disease-specific survival was seen as in younger populations; however, non–disease-related or non–treatment-related deaths were proportionally higher. No differences were seen in treatment-related toxicity, including hospitalization and treatment-related death. The authors concluded that although further study should be conducted in patients over the age of 75, adjuvant chemotherapy for resected NSCLC should not be withheld on the basis of age [51].

It is unlikely that a clinical trial specifically evaluating adjuvant chemotherapy or radiotherapy in elderly patients with resected N2 NSCLC will be conducted. Investigators and clinicians are left with retrospective and subset analyses, which provide little in the way of definitive evidence. Increased accrual of elderly patients into future clinical trials is imperative.

Future directions

Although adjuvant chemotherapy improves survival after resection of NSCLC with N2 disease, the administration of systemic therapy in the postoperative setting can prove difficult. Because patients have a better performance status before surgical resection, it has been argued that preoperative chemotherapy may be easier to administer to a larger percentage of patients. Smaller phase III clinical trials have indicated a survival benefit with neoadjuvant chemotherapy followed by surgical resection in NSCLC [52,53]; unfortunately, larger trials have yet to confirm this benefit [54–56]. The evidence and potential roles of neoadjuvant therapy are addressed in detail in another article in this issue. To date, evidence directly comparing the two treatment approaches is lacking. The NATCH trial is an ongoing large randomized trial comparing neoadjuvant systemic chemotherapy with adjuvant chemotherapy for resectable NSCLC (N2 disease is not included in this trial). More than 600 patients are randomized, and survival data are expected to become available within the next year [57]. It remains to be seen whether neoadjuvant chemotherapy may have a similar survival benefit.

The addition of newer "targeted agents" to standard chemotherapy has promised hope in improving on a therapeutic plateau that has been reached with systemic chemotherapy alone. Bevacizumab (Avastin), a monoclonal antibody targeted against vascular endothelial growth factor, has demonstrated survival benefit in patients with metastatic NSCLC [58]. This finding has prompted further evaluation of the combination of bevacizumab with chemotherapy in the adjuvant setting for NSCLC. The ECOG 1505 study is a phase III trial randomizing patients with resected stage IB-IIIA NSCLC to receive cisplatin-based adjuvant chemotherapy with or without bevacizumab [59]. The study is being conducted through the Intergroup. Survival information from this currently accruing trial will not be available for years.

Stimulation of the host immune system to recognize and fight cancer has intrigued researchers for decades. The melanoma-associated antigens (MAGE) are part of a family of tumor-associated antigens. The subtype MAGE-A3 antigen is expressed in approximately 35% of early-stage lung cancers [60]. In a randomized placebo-controlled phase II study involving 180 patients with resected stage IB and II NSCLC whose tumors expressed MAGE-A3, a 33% improvement in the disease-free interval was demonstrated with the MAGE-A3 vaccine (hazard ratio 0.67; $P = .121$) [61]. Currently, a randomized phase III trial of resected stages IB-IIIA NSCLC expressing MAGE-A3 gene is accruing patients. Patients will be stratified according to prior administration of platinum-based chemotherapy and will be randomized to receive the MAGE-A3 vaccine versus placebo [59]. Other vaccines are in varying stages of development and evaluation in NSCLC, but the MAGE-A3 vaccine is the most advanced in clinical testing currently.

Not all patients who are administered adjuvant chemotherapy benefit from the agents. Although recurrence rates after resection of NSCLC are high, especially with N2 involvement, some patients do not harbor micrometastatic disease and may be cured with surgery alone. Other patients experience disease recurrence despite the administration of adjuvant therapy at the expense of experiencing potentially life-threatening adverse effects of the treatment.

Identifying patients and tumors that may benefit from, or be resistant to, adjuvant chemotherapy at the time of diagnosis or resection may allow for chemotherapy to be tailored for maximal benefit. The excision repair cross-complementation group 1 (ERCC1) enzyme is a DNA repair enzyme associated with cisplatin resistance [62]. In a substudy of IALT (the IALT Bio study), ERCC1 expression was evaluated by immunohistochemical analysis, and the expression was correlated with survival outcomes [63]. ERCC1 expression was positive in 44% of the 761 tumors evaluable. Lack of ERCC1 expression was associated with a survival benefit with adjuvant chemotherapy (hazard ratio of death 0.65; $P = .002$). ERCC1-positive tumors did not experience a survival benefit with adjuvant chemotherapy (hazard ratio of death 1.41; $P = .40$). ERCC1 expression was associated with longer survival in patients who did not receive chemotherapy compared with patients who had ERCC1-negative tumors and did not receive chemotherapy (hazard ratio for death 0.66; $P = .009$). The authors concluded that patients with ERCC1-negative tumors benefited from adjuvant cisplatin-based chemotherapy, whereas patients with ERCC1-positive tumors did not [63].

The ribonucleoside reductase gene (RRM1) is the molecular target of gemcitabine chemotherapy. High levels of RRM1 expression in NSCLC have been correlated in a phase II study of 40 patients with previously untreated locally advanced NSCLC with an inverse response to gemcitabine chemotherapy ($P = .002$) [64]. In another series of 187 patients with resected NSCLC who did not receive chemotherapy, high expression of RRM1 was associated with prolonged survival compared to low RRM1 expression (median overall survival >120 months with high RRM1 versus 60.2 months with low RRM1; hazard ratio for death 0.61; $P = .02$) [65]. The combination of high ERCC1 and high RRM1 expression was associated with a survival advantage. Evaluation of ERCC1 and RRM1 expression has been applied to tailor therapy in a feasibility trial of patients with advanced NSCLC, and a confirmatory phase III trial is ongoing [66]. Should the analysis of molecular expression prove to have a survival advantage in tailoring chemotherapy, the next step would be evaluation in the adjuvant setting.

Summary

Since the publication of the meta-analysis in 1995 indicating a potential survival benefit with adjuvant cisplatin-based chemotherapy for patients with resected NSCLC, the management of patients with resected NSCLC and N2 disease involvement has evolved dramatically. The delivery of systemic therapy in the postoperative setting remains difficult, however, because tolerance for the toxicities of chemotherapy is reduced by recovery from surgery itself. Even with a proven survival benefit with adjuvant chemotherapy, cure is not guaranteed, and most patients die from relapse of their cancer. Optimization of treatment through the administration of neoadjuvant therapy, application of more modern radiotherapy techniques, and combined-modality therapy with chemoradiation or molecularly targeted agents are areas currently under active investigation. Ideally, the improvement of prediction of which patients harbor micrometastatic disease before undergoing surgical resection and the prediction of which patients would benefit from different systemic therapies may help to improve further the chance of cure for NSCLC while at the same time reducing toxicity.

References

[1] Jemal A, Siegel R, Ward E, et al. Cancer statistics, 2007. CA Cancer J Clin 2007;57:43–66.

[2] Kamangar F, Dores GM, Anderson WF. Patterns of cancer incidence, mortality, and prevalence across five continents: defining priorities to reduce cancer disparities in different geographic regions of the world. J Clin Oncol 2006;24:2137–50.

[3] Owonikoko TK, Ragin CC, Belani CP, et al. Lung cancer in elderly patients: an analysis of the Surveillance, Epidemiology, and End Results database. J Clin Oncol 2007;25:5570–7.

[4] Lee PC, Port JL, Korst RJ, et al. Risk factors for occult mediastinal metastases in clinical stage I non-small cell lung cancer. Ann Thorac Surg 2007;84:177–81.

[5] Douillard J-Y, Rosell R, De Lena M, et al. Impact of postoperative radiation therapy on survival in patients with complete resection and stage I, II, or IIIA non-small-cell lung cancer treated with adjuvant chemotherapy: the Adjuvant Navelbine International Trialist Association (ANITA) randomized trial. Int J Radiat Oncol Biol Phys 2008; [PUBLISHED AHEAD OF PRINT].

[6] Andre F, Grunenwald D, Pignon J-P, et al. Survival of patients with resected N2 non-small-cell lung cancer: evidence for a subclassification and implications. J Clin Oncol 2000;18:2981–9.

[7] Albain KS, Swann RS, Rusch VR, et al. Phase III study of concurrent chemotherapy and radiotherapy vs CT/RT followed by surgical resection for stage IIIA (pN2) non-small cell lung cancer: outcomes update of North American Intergroup 0139 (RTOG 9309) [abstract]. Proc Am Soc Clin Oncol 2005;23:7014.

[8] Pieterman RM, van Putten JWG, Meuzelaar JJ, et al. Preoperative staging of non-small-cell lung cancer with positron-emission tomography. N Engl J Med 2000;343:254–61.

[9] Hara M, Shiraki N, Itoh M, et al. A problem in diagnosing N3 disease using FDG-PET in patients with lung cancer: high false positive rate with visual assessment. Ann Nucl Med 2004;18:484–8.

[10] Shim SS, Lee KS, Kim B-T, et al. Focal parenchymal lung lesions showing a potential of false-positive and false-negative interpretations on integrated PET/CT. Am J Roentgenol 2006;186:639–48.

[11] Ohtsuka T, Nomori H, Watanabe K, et al. False-positive findings on [^{18}F]FDG-PET caused by non-neoplastic cellular elements after neoadjuvant chemoradiotherapy for non-small cell lung cancer. Jpn J Clin Oncol 2005;35:271–3.

[12] Silvestri GA, Gould MK, Margolis ML, et al. Non-invasive staging of non-small cell lung cancer: ACCP evidenced-based clinical practice guidelines (2nd edition). Chest 2007;132:178S–201S.

[13] Tournoy KG, De Ryck F, Vanwalleghem LR, et al. Endoscopic ultrasound reduces surgical mediastinal staging in lung cancer: a randomized trial. Am J Respir Crit Care Med 2008;177:531–5.

[14] Wallace MB, Pascual JMS, Raimondo M, et al. Minimally invasive endoscopic staging of suspected lung cancer. JAMA 2008;299:540–6.

[15] Non-Small-Cell Lung Cancer Collaborative Group. Chemotherapy in non-small cell lung cancer: a meta-analysis using updated data on individual patients from 52 randomised clinical trials. BMJ 1995;311:899–909.

[16] Arriagada R, Bergman B, Dunant A, et al. Cisplatin-based adjuvant chemotherapy in patients with completely resected non-small-cell lung cancer. N Engl J Med 2004;350:351–60.

[17] Le Chevalier T, Dunant A, Arriagada R, et al. Long-term results of the International Adjuvant Lung Cancer Trial (IALT) evaluating adjuvant cisplatin-based chemotherapy in resected non-small cell lung cancer [abstract]. Proc Am Soc Clin Oncol 2008;26:7507.

[18] Douillard J-Y, Rosell R, De Lena M, et al. Adjuvant vinorelbine plus cisplatin versus observation in patients with completely resected stage IB-IIIA non-small-cell lung cancer (Adjuvant Navelbine International Trialist Association [ANITA]): a randomised controlled trial. Lancet Oncol 2006;7:719–27.

[19] Scagliotti GV, Fossati R, Torri V, et al. Adjuvant Lung Project Italy/European Organisation for Research Treatment of Cancer-Lung Cancer Cooperative Group Investigators. Randomized study of adjuvant chemotherapy for completely resected stage I, II, or IIIA non-small-cell lung cancer. J Natl Cancer Inst 2003;95:1453–61.

[20] Waller D, Peake MD, Stephens RJ, et al. Chemotherapy for patients with non-small cell lung cancer: the surgical setting of the Big Lung Trial. Eur J Cardiothorac Surg 2004;26:173–82.

[21] Pignon JP, Tribodet H, Scagliotti GV, et al. Lung Adjuvant Cisplatin Evaluation (LACE): a pooled analysis of five randomized clinical trials including 4,584 patients [abstract]. Proc Am Soc Clin Oncol 2006;24:7008.

[22] The Study Group of Adjuvant Chemotherapy for Lung Cancer (Chubu, Japan). A randomized trial of postoperative adjuvant chemotherapy in non-small cell lung cancer (the second cooperative study). Eur J Surg Oncol 1995;21:69–77.

[23] Wada H, Hitomi S, Teramatsu T, et al. Adjuvant chemotherapy after complete resection in non-small-cell lung cancer. J Clin Oncol 1996;14:1048–54.

[24] Nakagawa K, Tada H, Akashi A, et al. Randomised study of adjuvant chemotherapy for completely resected p-stage I-IIIA non-small cell lung cancer. Br J Cancer 2006;95:817–21.

[25] Tanaka F, Tsubota N, Namikawa S, et al. A randomized phase III trial of adjuvant chemotherapy with cisplatin and vindesine followed by UFT for completely resected pathologic stage IIIA-N2 non-small cell lung cancer: West Japan Study Group for Lung Cancer Surgery (WJSG), the 5th study [abstract]. Proc Am Soc Clin Oncol 2005;23:7262.

[26] Hamada C, Tanaka F, Ohta M, et al. Meta-analysis of postoperative adjuvant chemotherapy with tegafur-uracil in non-small-cell lung cancer. J Clin Oncol 2005;23:4999–5006.

[27] Stewart LA, Burdett S, Tierney JF, et al. Surgery and adjuvant chemotherapy compared to surgery alone in non-small cell lung cancer: a meta-analysis using individual patient data from randomized clinical trials [abstract]. Proc Am Soc Clin Oncol 2007;25:7552.

[28] PORT Meta-Analysis Trialists Group. Postoperative radiotherapy in non-small-cell lung cancer: systematic review and meta-analysis of individual patient data from nine randomised controlled trials. Lancet 1998;352:257–63.

[29] Burdett S, Stewart L, PORT Meta-analysis Group. Postoperative radiotherapy in non-small-cell lung cancer: update of an individual patient data meta-analysis. Lung Cancer 2005;47:81–3.

[30] Bonner JA. The role of postoperative radiotherapy for patients with completely resected nonsmall cell lung carcinoma: seeking to optimize local control and survival while minimizing toxicity. Cancer 1999;86:195–6.

[31] Machtay M, Kaiser LR, Glatstein E. Reality and meta-analyses. Chest 2000;118:835–6.

[32] Marks LB, Prosnitz LR. Postoperative radiotherapy for lung cancer: the breast cancer story all over again? Int J Radiat Oncol Biol Phys 2000;48:625–7.

[33] Munro AJ. What now for postoperative radiotherapy for lung cancer? Lancet 1998;352:250–1.

[34] Bogart JA, Aronowitz JN. Localized non-small cell lung cancer: adjuvant radiotherapy in the era of effective systemic therapy. Clin Cancer Res 2005;11:5004S–10S.

[35] Phlips P, Rocmans P, Vanderhoeft P, et al. Postoperative radiotherapy after pneumonectomy: impact of modern treatment facilities. Int J Radiat Oncol Biol Phys 1993;27:525–9.

[36] Roach M 3rd, Gandara DR, You HS, et al. Radiation pneumonitis following combined modality

therapy for lung cancer: analysis of prognostic factors. J Clin Oncol 1995;13:2606–12.
[37] Lally BE, Zelterman D, Colasanto JM, et al. Postoperative radiotherapy for stage II or III non-small-cell lung cancer using the Surveillance, Epidemiology, and End Results database. J Clin Oncol 2006;24: 2998–3006.
[38] Lally BE, Detterbeck FC, Geiger AM, et al. The risk of death from heart disease in patients with nonsmall cell lung cancer who receive postoperative radiotherapy: analysis of the Surveillance, Epidemiology, and End Results database. Cancer 2007;110: 911–7.
[39] Le Pechoux C, Dunant A, Pignon J-P. Need for a new trial to evaluate adjuvant postoperative radiotherapy in non-small-cell lung cancer patients with N2 mediastinal involvement. J Clin Oncol 2007;25: e10–11.
[40] Pisters KMW, Evans WK, Azzoli CG, et al. Cancer Care Ontario and American Society of Clinical Oncology adjuvant chemotherapy and adjuvant radiation therapy for stages I-IIIA resectable non-small-cell lung cancer guideline. J Clin Oncol 2007; 25:5506–18.
[41] Robinson LA, Ruckdeschel JC, Wagner H Jr, et al. Treatment of non-small cell lung cancer, stage IIIA: ACCP evidence-based clinical practice guidelines (2nd edition). Chest 2007;132:S243–65.
[42] Keller SM, Adak S, Wagner H, et al. A randomized trial of postoperative adjuvant therapy in patients with completely resected stage II or IIIA non-small-cell lung cancer. N Engl J Med 2000;343: 1217–22.
[43] Bradley JD, Paulus R, Graham MV, et al. Phase II trial of postoperative adjuvant paclitaxel/carboplatin and thoracic radiotherapy in resected stage II and IIIA non-small-cell lung cancer: promising long-term results of the Radiation Therapy Oncology Group—RTOG 9705. J Clin Oncol 2005;23: 3480–7.
[44] Greco FA, Burris HA III, Gray JR, et al. Paclitaxel and carboplatin adjuvant therapy alone or with radiotherapy for resected nonsmall cell lung carcinoma: a feasibility study of the Minnie Pearl Cancer Research Network. Cancer 2001;92:2142–7.
[45] Andre F, Grunenwald D, Pujol JL, et al. Patterns of relapse of N2 nonsmall-cell lung carcinoma patients treated with preoperative chemotherapy: should prophylactic cranial irradiation be reconsidered? Cancer 2001;91:2394–400.
[46] Mamon HJ, Yeap BY, Janne PA, et al. High risk of brain metastases in surgically staged IIIA non-small-cell lung cancer patients treated with surgery, chemotherapy, and radiation. J Clin Oncol 2005; 23:1530–7.
[47] Auperin A, Arriagada R, Pignon JP, et al. Prophylactic cranial irradiation for patients with small-cell lung cancer in complete remission. N Engl J Med 1999;341:476–84.
[48] Slotman B, Faivre-Finn C, Kramer G, et al. Prophylactic cranial irradiation in extensive small-cell lung cancer. N Engl J Med 2007;357:664–72.
[49] Available at: www.rtog.org Accessed May 8, 2008.
[50] Pottgen C, Eberhardt W, Grannass A, et al. Prophylactic cranial irradiation in operable stage IIIA non-small-cell lung cancer treated with neoadjuvant chemoradiotherapy: results from a German multicenter randomized trial. J Clin Oncol 2007;25:4987–92.
[51] Pepe C, Hasan B, Winton TL, et al. Adjuvant vinorelbine and cisplatin in elderly patients: National Cancer Institute of Canada and Intergroup Study JBR.10. J Clin Oncol 2007;25:1553–61.
[52] Roth JA, Fossella F, Komaki R, et al. A randomized trial comparing perioperative chemotherapy and surgery with surgery alone in resectable stage IIIA non-small cell lung cancer. J Natl Cancer Inst 1994;86:673–80.
[53] Rosell R, Gomez-Codina J, Camps C, et al. A randomized trial comparing preoperative chemotherapy plus surgery with surgery alone in patients with non-small-cell lung cancer. N Engl J Med 1994;330:153–8.
[54] Depierre A, Milleron B, Moro-Sibilot D, et al. Preoperative chemotherapy followed by surgery compared with primary surgery in resectable stage I (except T1N0), II, and IIIA non-small-cell lung cancer. J Clin Oncol 2002;20:247–53.
[55] Nagai K, Tsuchiya R, Mori T, et al. A randomized trial comparing induction chemotherapy followed by surgery with surgery alone for patients with stage IIIA N2 non-small cell lung cancer (JCOG 9209). J Thorac Cardiovasc Surg 2003;125:254–60.
[56] Gilligan D, Nicolson M, Smith I, et al. Preoperative chemotherapy in patients with resectable non-small cell lung cancer: results of the MRC LU22/NVALT 2/EORTC 08012 multicentre randomized trial and update of systematic review. Lancet 2007;369: 1929–37.
[57] Felip E, Rosell R, Massuti B, et al. The NATCH trial: observations on the neoadjuvant arm [abstract]. Proc Am Soc Clin Oncol 2007;25:7578.
[58] Sandler AB, Gray R, Perry MC, et al. Paclitaxel-carboplatin alone or with bevacizumab for non-small-cell lung cancer. N Engl J Med 2006;355:2542–50.
[59] Available at: www.clinicaltrials.gov Accessed June 19, 2008.
[60] Sienel W, Verwerk C, Linder A, et al. Melanoma associated antigen (MAGE)-A3 expression in stages I and II non-small cell lung cancer: results of a multi-center study. Eur J Cardiothorac Surg 2004;24:131–4.
[61] Vansteenkiste J, Zielinski M, Dahabre J, et al. Multicenter, double-blind, randomized, placebo-controlled phase II study to assess the efficacy of recombinant MAGE-A3 vaccine as adjuvant therapy in stage IB/II MAGE-A3-positive, completely resected, non-small cell lung cancer [abstract]. Proc Am Soc Clin Oncol 2006;24:7019.

[62] Lord RV, Brabender J, Gandara D, et al. Low ERCC1 expression correlates with prolonged survival after cisplatin plus gemcitabine chemotherapy in non-small cell lung cancer. Clin Cancer Res 2002;8:2286–91.

[63] Olaussen KA, Dunant A, Fouret P, et al. DNA repair by ERCC1 in non-small-cell lung cancer and cisplatin-based adjuvant chemotherapy. N Engl J Med 2006;355:983–91.

[64] Bepler G, Kusmartseva I, Sharma S, et al. *RRM1* modulated in vitro and in vivo efficacy of gemcitabine and platinum in non-small-cell lung cancer. J Clin Oncol 2006;24:4731–7.

[65] Zheng Z, Chen T, Li X, et al. DNA synthesis and repair genes *RRM1* and *ERCC1* in lung cancer. N Engl J Med 2007;356:800–8.

[66] Simon GR, Williams CC, Chiappori AA, et al. Molecular analysis-directed individualized therapy (MADeIT) in advanced non-small cell lung cancer [abstract]. Proc Am Soc Clin Oncol 2007;25: 7502.

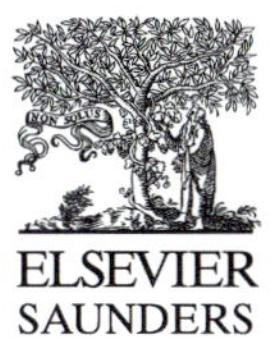

ELSEVIER
SAUNDERS

Thorac Surg Clin 18 (2008) 437–441

THORACIC
SURGERY
CLINICS

Management Algorithms for Stage IIIA Non–Small Cell Lung Cancer with N2 Node Involvement

Frank Detterbeck, MD[a,*], Mithran S. Sukumar, MD[b]

[a]*Department of Surgery, Section of Thoracic Surgery, Yale University, 333 Cedar Street, FMB 128, P.O. Box 208062, New Haven, CT 06520, USA*
[b]*Oregon Health Sciences University, Portland VA Medical Center, 3181 SW Sam Jackson Park Road, Portland, OR 97239, USA*

Stage IIIA non–small cell lung cancer (NSCLC) with N2 node involvement (IIIA[N2]) is a complex area characterized by much confusion and controversy. A major source of confusion is that data derived from a particular subgroup of IIIA(N2) often are inappropriately applied to another subgroup. The problem is not so much that stage IIIA(N2) encompasses a spectrum of disease, which is true in each stage of NSCLC. Rather, our ability to describe a patient cohort has been limited, and it is therefore often difficult to determine how and when to apply data from published studies.

A simple, pragmatic approach is taken in this article to define algorithms for the management of these patients. The simplicity of the algorithms represents both the strength of the article and its major weakness. Many nuances are important, and existing data may be interpreted from different viewpoints. A full discussion of all of these issues is not possible here, but the accompanying paragraphs touch on some of the major areas of consensus and controversy. The reader is directed to the references and other articles in this issue for further details. Ideally, one should critically discuss the management of these patients with other disciplines involved in one's local community, taking care not to extrapolate inappropriately from one cohort of patients to another.

Evaluation/staging of the mediastinum in patients who have non–small cell lung cancer

Patients who have NSCLC and potential mediastinal involvement can be divided into four distinct groups based on imaging studies [1]. This information is readily available and provides a guide as to how further imaging and invasive staging should be done [2]. Radiographic staging of the mediastinum is generally not accurate enough to proceed with recommendations for therapy unless mediastinal invasion or a peripheral clinical stage I (cI) tumor is obvious. Even a negative positron emission tomography in the mediastinum carries a high false-negative rate in many situations (Fig. 1) [2,3].

Mediastinal infiltration

Patients who have mediastinal infiltration, defined as N2 or N3 nodal enlargement that cannot be distinguished from a mass invading the mediastinum, can be treated definitively with intent to cure if they have a good performance status. The approach should be concurrent chemoradiotherapy. Patients who are not in good condition should receive palliative therapy and supportive care [4]. Palliative radiotherapy is recommended for actual symptoms; prophylactic palliative treatment is not supported by existing data (Fig. 2).

Clinical N2 nodal disease

Patients who have cytologically or histologically confirmed N2 involvement and are in good

* Corresponding author.
E-mail address: frank.detterbeck@yale.edu (F. Detterbeck).

doi:10.1016/j.thorsurg.2008.08.006

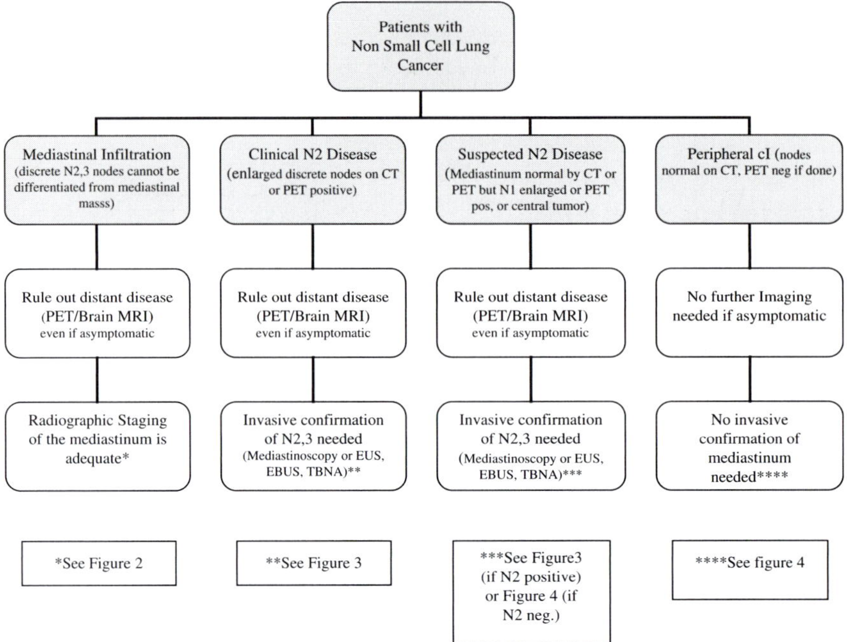

Fig. 1. Evaluation/staging of patients who have NSCLC with respect to categorization of the mediastinum. CT, computed tomography; EUS, esophageal ultrasound; MRI, magnetic resonance imaging; neg, negative; PET, positron emission tomography; pos, positive; TBNA, transbronchial needle aspiration.

condition should be treated with curative intent. The standard of care is concurrent chemoradiotherapy [4,5]. A reasonable alternative strategy is either a more aggressive bimodality approach (higher-dose radiotherapy, newer chemotherapy regimens) or a trimodality approach. Such treatment approaches should be done in the context of a clinical trial, or at the very least, as part of a written, prospective, fully defined policy of treatment, including patient selection, evaluation policies, and treatment plan. Much uncertainty surrounds the treatment of stage IIIA(N2) patients, and the local ability to provide certain aspects of the treatment can vary significantly (experience with imaging and invasive staging tests; surgical, radiotherapy and chemotherapy experience; facilities; and so forth.). A multidisciplinary working group to define an appropriate local policy prospectively is a minimum requirement if deviation from standard bimodality treatment is considered (Fig. 3) [4,5].

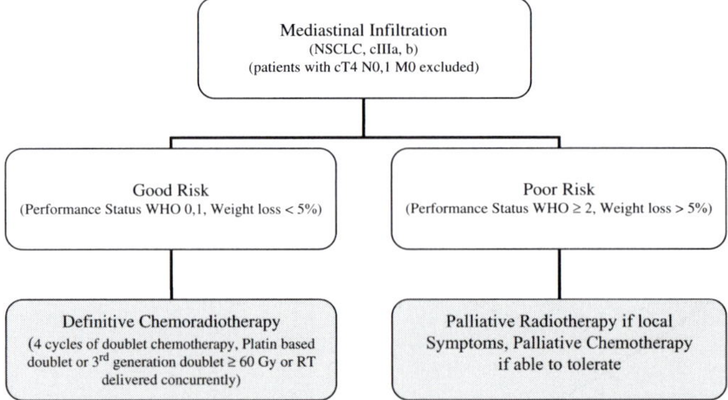

Fig. 2. Treatment of patients who have cIIIA,B NSCLC with mediastinal infiltration. cT4; Gy, gray; RT, radiotherapy; WHO, World Health Organization.

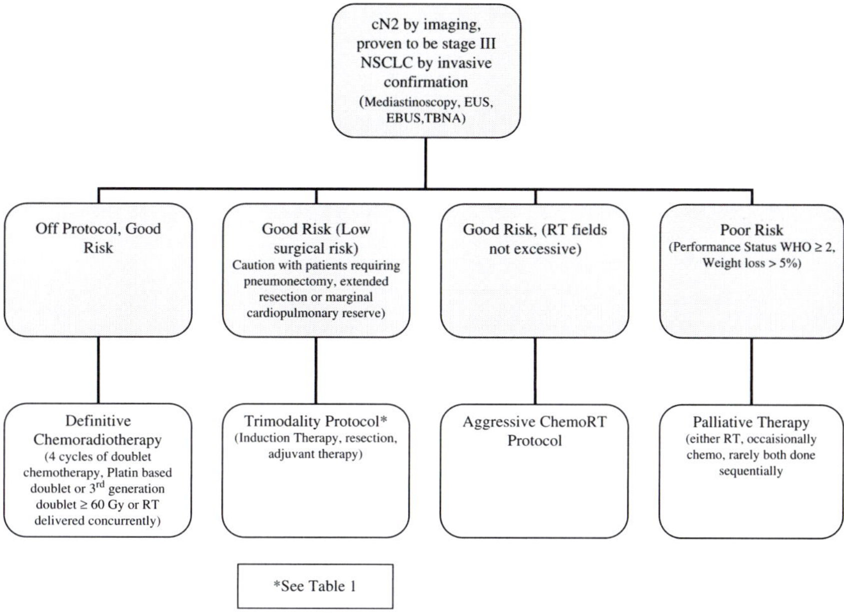

Fig. 3. Treatment of patients who have IIIA NSCLC with clinical N2 nodes.

Clinical N0,1 disease

If N2 disease is unexpectedly encountered intraoperatively in patients who have been carefully staged preoperatively, proceeding with resection is justified unless it is clear that a complete resection cannot be achieved [5,6]. Postoperative (adjuvant) chemotherapy is clearly indicated in such patients after resection. Whether radiotherapy should also be given is controversial (Fig. 4) [5,7].

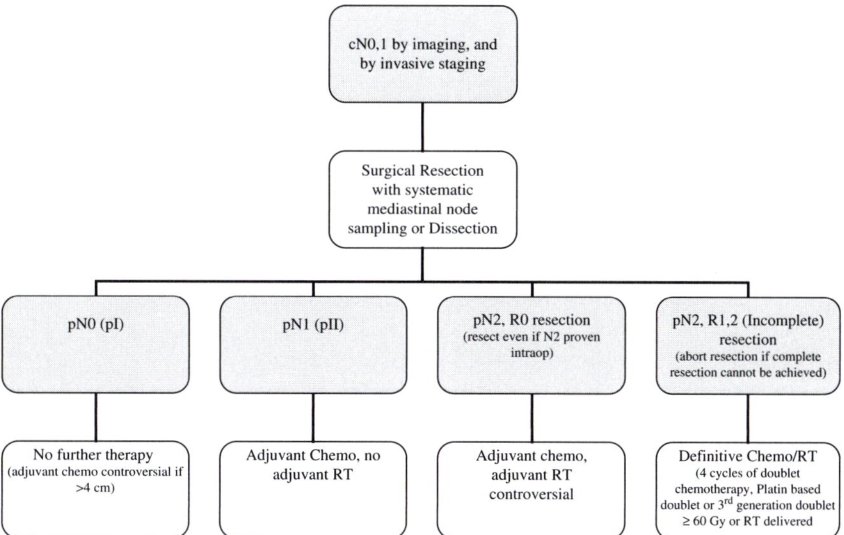

Fig. 4. Treatment of patients who have cN0,1 tumors. Chemo/RT, chemoradiotherapy; Gy, gray; p, pathologic; R, residual; RT, radiotherapy.

Trimodality therapy

Although a trimodality approach (chemotherapy, radiation, and surgery) is a commonly practiced treatment strategy for patients who have stage IIIA(N2) disease, almost every aspect of this approach is characterized more by unanswered questions than by data. Therefore, if this approach is to be used, it should be in the context of a clinical trial so we do not perpetually practice "by the seat of our pants" [5]. Table 1 points out the issues associated with each of the steps encountered in a typical trimodality approach. In addition, whether trimodality treatment is more beneficial than bimodality treatment (chemoradiotherapy) is controversial [8] (see Table 1).

Patient selection for trimodality treatment is a major issue. Most of the phase II studies of trimodality treatment have involved patients who had bulky and often multistation disease. Currently, however, the trend is toward selecting only patients who have minimal N2 disease (either small nodes or single station positive), despite the absence of data that this cohort is better served by tri- versus bimodality treatment. It is true that patients who have minimal N2 disease have a better prognosis, but this finding appears to be the case regardless of the treatment strategy used.

After induction therapy, a common practice is to restage patients to select those who have a better prognosis. One problem is the lack of a reliable method of restaging other than a primary (rather than a repeat) mediastinoscopy [3]. Furthermore, all of the data indicating that "downstaged" patients have a better prognosis come from series in which all patients were resected, thus defining who was downstaged. A particularly questionable

Table 1
Trimodality management of IIIA(N2) lung cancer

Treatment steps	Issue	Problem
Stage IIIA(N2) NSCLC	Patient selection: only those who have "minimal" N2 disease if single station positive?	No data support that these patients do better with trimodality than another approach. Most phase II and III trimodality studies included patients who had bulky N2 disease.
Induction therapy	Chemotherapy versus chemoradiotherapy	No clear data define one as superior.
	Best radiotherapy dose, chemotherapy regimen?	No clear data define one as superior.
Restaging	Define patients who have mediastinal downstaging	No reliable method exists of restaging except primary mediastinoscopy. (EUS, EBUS, remediastinoscopy, PET all have high false-negative rate.)
Persistent N2 (cyN2)	Are persistent N2 the patients who should not be resected because of a poor response, or who should be resected because of poor response to induction therapy?	No data are available to answer this question.
Downstaged (cyN0,1)	Are downstaged patients the ones who should be resected because of a good response, or those who should not be resected because of a good response to induction therapy?	No data are available to answer this question.
Resection and node dissection	Perioperative mortality	Perioperative mortality may easily offset any oncologic benefit.
	Resect originally involved tissues or perform a lesser resection?	No data exist to support a lesser resection.
Adjuvant therapy	Chemotherapy?	Well-supported data exist for IIIA(N2) patients who have not had induction treatment; they are less clear in the setting of induction treatment.
	Radiotherapy?	Controversial.

approach is to use the response as seen by chest CT to select patients. Extensive data indicate that shrinkage has poor correlation with the presence or absence of viable tumor in the mediastinum when resection on all patients is performed. Finally, although it is clear that responders do better, this prognostic information does not define the benefit of surgical resection. Interruption of treatment for purposes of restaging has the potential downside of compromising the effectiveness of chemoradiotherapy if a decision is made not to perform resection. In summary, the concept of restaging is problematic because of a lack of reliable methods of restaging, and a lack of data showing that restaging is a legitimate method to determine who will benefit from a tri- versus a bimodality strategy (although they do provide prognostic information).

A trimodality treatment approach should be done in the context of a clinical trial, or at the very least, a written, prospective plan defining the selection, evaluation, and treatment, developed by a local multidisciplinary group with expertise in treating NSCLC.

References

[1] Silvestri G, Gould MK, Margolis ML, et al. Non-invasive staging of non-small cell lung cancer: ACCP evidenced-based clinical practice guidelines. 2nd edition. Chest 2007;132(3 Suppl):178S–201S.

[2] Detterbeck F, Jantz M, Wallace M, et al. Invasive mediastinal staging of lung cancer: an ACCP evidence based clinical practice guidelines (2nd edition). Chest 2007;132(3 Suppl):202S–20S.

[3] Detterbeck F. Integration of mediastinal staging techniques for lung cancer. Semin Thorac Cardiovasc Surg. 2007;19(3):217–24.

[4] Jett JR, Schild S, Keith R, et al. Treatment of non-small cell lung cancer–stage IIIB: ACCP evidenced-based clinical practice guidelines. Chest 2007;132 (3 Suppl):266S–276.

[5] Robinson L, Ruckdeschel J, Wagner HJ, et al. Treatment of non-small cell lung cancer–stage IIIA: ACCP evidence-based guidelines (2nd edition). Chest 2007; 132(3 Suppl):243S–65S.

[6] Detterbeck F. What to do with "surprise" N2: intraoperative management of patients with non-small cell lung cancer. J Thorac Oncol 2008;7: 781–92.

[7] Lally BE, Zelterman D, Colasanto JM, et al. Postoperative radiotherapy for stage II or III non-small-cell lung cancer using the surveillance, epidemiology, and end results database. J Clin Oncol. 2006;24(19): 2998–3006.

[8] West H, Albain K. Current standards and ongoing controversies in the management of locally advanced non-small cell lung cancer. Semin Oncol 2005;32(3): 284–92.

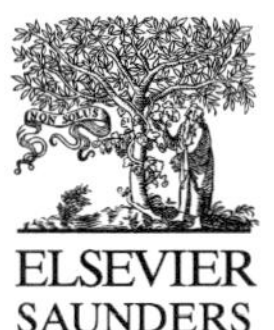
ELSEVIER
SAUNDERS

Thorac Surg Clin 18 (2008) 443–447

THORACIC SURGERY CLINICS

Index

Note: Page numbers of article titles are in **boldface** type.

1547-4127/08/$ - see front matter
doi:10.1016/S1547-4127(08)00099-6

P

R

S

T

U

V

X

United States Postal Service

Statement of Ownership, Management, and Circulation (All Periodicals Publications Except Requestor Publications)

1. Publication Title	2. Publication Number	3. Filing Date
Thoracic Surgery Clinics	0 1 3 - 1 2 6	9/15/08
4. Issue Frequency Feb, May, Aug, Nov	5. Number of Issues Published Annually 4	6. Annual Subscription Price $220.00

7. Complete Mailing Address of Known Office of Publication (*Not printer*) (*Street, city, county, state, and ZIP+4*)

Elsevier Inc.
360 Park Avenue South
New York, NY 10010-1710

Contact Person: Stephen Bushing
Telephone (Include area code): 215-239-3688

8. Complete Mailing Address of Headquarters or General Business Office of Publisher (*Not printer*)

Elsevier Inc., 360 Park Avenue South, New York, NY 10010-1710

9. Full Names and Complete Mailing Addresses of Publisher, Editor, and Managing Editor (*Do not leave blank*)

Publisher (*Name and complete mailing address*)

John Schrefer , Elsevier, Inc., 1600 John F. Kennedy Blvd. Suite 1800, Philadelphia, PA 19103-2899

Editor (*Name and complete mailing address*)

Catherine Bewick, Elsevier, Inc., 1600 John F. Kennedy Blvd. Suite 1800, Philadelphia, PA 19103-2899

Managing Editor (*Name and complete mailing address*)

Catherine Bewick, Elsevier, Inc., 1600 John F. Kennedy Blvd. Suite 1800, Philadelphia, PA 19103-2899

10. Owner (*Do not leave blank. If the publication is owned by a corporation, give the name and address of the corporation immediately followed by the names and addresses of all stockholders owning or holding 1 percent or more of the total amount of stock. If not owned by a corporation, give the names and addresses of the individual owners. If owned by a partnership or other unincorporated firm, give its name and address as well as those of each individual owner. If the publication is published by a nonprofit organization, give its name and address.*)

Full Name	Complete Mailing Address
Wholly owned subsidiary of	4520 East-West Highway
Reed/Elsevier, US holdings	Bethesda, MD 20814

11. Known Bondholders, Mortgagees, and Other Security Holders Owning or Holding 1 Percent or More of Total Amount of Bonds, Mortgages, or Other Securities. If none, check box → ☐ None

Full Name	Complete Mailing Address
N/A	

12. Tax Status (*For completion by nonprofit organizations authorized to mail at nonprofit rates*) (*Check one*)
The purpose, function, and nonprofit status of this organization and the exempt status for federal income tax purposes:
☐ Has Not Changed During Preceding 12 Months
☐ Has Changed During Preceding 12 Months (*Publisher must submit explanation of change with this statement*)

PS Form 3526, September 2006 (Page 1 of 3 (Instructions Page 3)) PSN 7530-01-000-9931 **PRIVACY NOTICE**: See our Privacy policy in www.usps.com

13. Publication Title: Thoracic Surgery Clinics

14. Issue Date for Circulation Data Below: August 2008

15. Extent and Nature of Circulation			Average No. Copies Each Issue During Preceding 12 Months	No. Copies of Single Issue Published Nearest to Filing Date
a. Total Number of Copies (*Net press run*)			1775	1500
b. Paid Circulation (By Mail and Outside the Mail)	(1)	Mailed Outside-County Paid Subscriptions Stated on PS Form 3541. (*Include paid distribution above nominal rate, advertiser's proof copies, and exchange copies*)	721	677
	(2)	Mailed In-County Paid Subscriptions Stated on PS Form 3541 (*Include paid distribution above nominal rate, advertiser's proof copies, and exchange copies*)		
	(3)	Paid Distribution Outside the Mails Including Sales Through Dealers and Carriers, Street Vendors, Counter Sales, and Other Paid Distribution Outside USPS®	362	375
	(4)	Paid Distribution by Other Classes Mailed Through the USPS (e.g. First-Class Mail®)		
c. Total Paid Distribution (*Sum of 15b (1), (2), (3), and (4)*) ►			1083	1052
d. Free or Nominal Rate Distribution (By Mail and Outside the Mail)	(1)	Free or Nominal Rate Outside-County Copies Included on PS Form 3541	52	50
	(2)	Free or Nominal Rate In-County Copies Included on PS Form 3541		
	(3)	Free or Nominal Rate Copies Mailed at Other Classes Mailed Through the USPS (e.g. First-Class Mail)		
	(4)	Free or Nominal Rate Distribution Outside the Mail (Carriers or other means)		
e. Total Free or Nominal Rate Distribution (Sum of 15d (1), (2), (3) and (4)			52	50
f. Total Distribution (Sum of 15c and 15e) ►			1135	1102
g. Copies not Distributed (See instructions to publishers #4 (page #3)) ►			640	398
h. Total (Sum of 15f and g)			1775	1500
i. Percent Paid (15c divided by 15f times 100) ►			95.42%	95.46%

16. Publication of Statement of Ownership

☐ If the publication is a general publication, publication of this statement is required. Will be printed in the **November 2008** issue of this publication. ☐ Publication not required

17. Signature and Title of Editor, Publisher, Business Manager, or Owner

Jean Fanucci – Executive Director of Subscription Services

Date: September 15, 2008

I certify that all information furnished on this form is true and complete. I understand that anyone who furnishes false or misleading information on this form or who omits material or information requested on the form may be subject to criminal sanctions (including fines and imprisonment) and/or civil sanctions (including civil penalties).

PS Form 3526, September 2006 (Page 2 of 3)